MOVING THROUGH MENOPAUSE WITH GRACE:

A Stress-free Guide to Finding Your New Normal Less Pain, Improved Sleep, and Emotional Balance

LAURIE MORSE, L.AC.

TABLE OF CONTENTS

INTRODUCTION

Menopause is often whispered about in hushed tones, shrouded in mystery and misconceptions, and painted as a time of loss—of youth, beauty, and vitality. But what if I told you that menopause could be one of the most empowering, clarifying, and transformative experiences of your life? What if, instead of fearing it, you could embrace this phase with an anticipation of peace, self-discovery, and restoration of spirit that radiates from within? This is not just a possibility; it's a promise I extend to you as we step into this journey together.

"I wish we were more open about the menopause - I've been in absolute bits at times."

— AMANDA REDMAN

My work with Chinese Medicine for over three decades has taught me a deep understanding of the intricate balance between body, mind, and spirit. As a Sacred Health Mentor and the author of works that have guided women through the ebbs and flows of heart health, menopause, and stress management, my path has been one of bridging the ancient wisdom of the East with the scientific advancements of the West. This book is the culmination of years spent walking alongside women like you through the fires of transformation that menopause brings.

Moving through Menopause with Grace: A Stress-Free Guide to Finding Your New Normal is your compass in navigating the sometimes-tumultuous waters of menopause. It's crafted to bring you mental, emotional, physical, and spiritual support as you traverse the stages of perimenopause, menopause, and postmenopausal. With a language that calms your mind, speaks to your soul, and practical steps that ground you in your daily life, this book is your invitation to a journey of healing, discovery, and rebirth.

As we turn these pages together, you'll find a tapestry of personal anecdotes, case studies, and the gentle guidance of someone who has not only researched but lived and breathed the teachings of this book. This is a general guidebook, not a tome, as that would be too big! This guidebook is designed to get you started and to help you move from where you are to where you want to be. From integrating Chinese medicine and personal energy management to embracing your Sacred Self, our exploration will be as diverse as it is deep.

You, dear reader, are not alone. Within these pages lies a community, a sisterhood of souls ready to support and uplift you through this transformation. We'll debunk myths, face fears, and emerge on the other side with a newfound appreciation for the beauty and wisdom that menopause brings.

You can skim the basic information if you're farther along the path. If you're new to the path, take it all in. No matter where you are on your journey, please read the last chapter, where I get real and raw.

I'll also point out that the deliberate repetition in this book is due to the inherent nature of our human minds. This intentional approach is based on the understanding that repetition is a fundamental requirement for effective learning and retention. If you're reading something for the second or third time and it's making you crazy, just move along.

This book is unique because it doesn't just focus on the physical aspect of menopause but dives into the soulful, creative, and spiritual awakening menopause can herald. It beckons us to rise, empowered and enlightened through the experience, coming out the other side more whole than before. Take what resonates, leave what doesn't.

I invite you now to step into this journey with me, with an open heart and mind, to embrace menopause not as the end but as the beginning of a vibrant, meaningful chapter of our lives. We will navigate this path armed with knowledge, supported by wisdom, and inspired by the new possibilities that await.

Every woman's life has a moment where the divine wholeness of life beckons, inviting her to step into her power, wisdom, and grace. Menopause is not just a transition; it's an awakening.

Let this be the moment you answer that call.

CHAPTER 1

THE LAY OF THE LAND

In the epic chrysalis of a woman's existence, there's a moment when age, hormones, wisdom, and change decide to throw a wild party, creating a phase that can only be described as "transformation with a side of tricky." This soiree, known as menopause, likes to make an entrance, complete with a mysterious tone and a few misconceptions hanging out in the corner.

This chrysalis is an unexpected and profound opportunity for deep personal growth, understanding, and self-awareness. Menopause isn't just Mother Nature hitting the pause button on the fertile phase; it's more like an exclusive VIP ticket to a sacred gathering where you get to know yourself better by learning to move with the rhythms of life. Who knew midlife could be this happening?

One last thing on this note... according to Star Trek... resistance is futile. A caterpillar can't get herself out of the chrysalis on the way to becoming a butterfly. She either moves through or perishes. I think that moving through with grace is the best option we have.

In this chapter, we'll look at the overview first.

1.1 THE SCIENCE AND SOUL OF MENOPAUSE: UNRAVELING THE MYSTERY

Amid the myriad of changes a woman undergoes throughout her life, menopause is a significant milestone. It signals the end of menstrual cycles but viewing it only through the lens of biology is a disservice. Menopause is as much a spiritual and emotional passage as it is a physical one.

Understanding Menopause

Menopause is defined by the conclusion of menstrual periods for twelve consecutive months. This definition, however, *barely scratches the surface* of what menopause embodies. The cessation of menstruation is a signal from the body that it is transitioning into a new phase, not governed by the monthly ebb and flow of eggs and hormones, but by a new rhythm altogether. This phase, often arriving sometime after age forty-five (unless surgically induced), is not an ailment but a natural biological process every woman experiences differently.

Biological and Spiritual Journey

The journey through menopause is a fusion of physical adjustments to changing hormone levels, brain pathways, and a deeper, more introspective journey. It's a period that invites women to reflect on their lives, bodies, and futures. As hormone levels shift, so does a woman's perspective on herself and her place in the world. This transition is an invitation to explore aspects of the self that may have been overshadowed by the demands of fertility and childbearing years. If you didn't have children, whether by choice or not, other demands likely overshadowed exploring more profound aspects of yourself.

Hormonal Changes

The hormonal orchestra that plays throughout a woman's life undergoes a significant shift during menopause. Estrogen and progesterone, hormones that have regulated menstruation and fertility, decrease significantly. This reduction impacts the reproductive system and has far-reaching effects on other bodily functions, influencing everything from brain function and bone density to cardiovascular health. Cortisol—often termed the stress hormone—testosterone and thyroid hormones can also fluctuate during this time, affecting a woman's mood, energy, and stress levels. Understanding these changes is crucial, not just for managing physical symptoms but for navigating the emotional and psychological landscape of menopause.

Embracing the Transition

The transition into menopause can often feel like uncharted waters, especially in the beginning. Once you realize it's happening and you get your sea legs, it becomes a time to reassess your health, relationships, life, and purpose. For many, it's a period of liberation from the fear of unwanted pregnancy, offering new freedom in sexual expression. Furthermore, the decrease in estrogen levels is not just a biological marker; it can be seen as shedding a layer, revealing the true core of a woman's being, untethered from her reproductive functions.

This phase also presents an opportunity to confront and redefine societal norms about aging and femininity. The prevailing narrative around menopause often focuses on the loss of youth, fertility,

and desirability. Yet this period can also be a time of great empowerment, a testament to women's resilience and strength.
Embracing menopause as a natural and essential phase of life
allows for a reconnection with the self, fostering a sense of inner
peace and wisdom that comes with age.

In the real world, this may mean a woman in her early fifties, grap-
pling with the initial signs of menopause, decides to take up yoga
or meditation—not just to manage hot flashes or sleep disturbances, but as a pathway to inner tranquility and self-acceptance.
She may also seek out communities or forums to share experiences and strategies, fostering a sense of connection and solidarity
with others navigating similar changes.

Some women cultivate creative expression as an outlet for
worries, emotions, and pain. During the most miserable part of
menopause, a creative part of me that I was utterly disconnected
from kept calling me, and I eventually listened (out of desperation!). Engaging in creativity became my lifeboat on the rough seas
of menopause, delivering me to shores of stability.

Through understanding and embracing the multifaceted nature of
menopause, women can transform this transition into a period of
renewal and empowerment. By recognizing the biological under-
pinnings of menopause and aligning them with a journey of spiritual and personal growth, the experience becomes not one of loss
but of profound discovery.

With guidance, this has been my experience and the experience of
just about all the women I know. But it didn't start that way!

I awoke one day in June at forty-two years old and felt like aliens
had taken over my body. I didn't recognize myself in any way,
shape, or form. Before then, there had been odd days here and

there, but it never felt like this. In hindsight, this was the moment menopause began, and I had no idea.

I assumed I'd sail through "the change" because I'm a healthcare professional and had been treating menopausal women for years; I recognized the profile. But I wasn't prepared for the terrain ahead.

Most women, in hindsight, recognize an increase in PMS, changing cycles, or more substantial mood swings and think, "Wow, my cycles seem more intense." Usually, when a menstrual cycle starts, PMS stops, but at some point, it doesn't stop—the intensity keeps going with seemingly no relief.

This was my experience for about seven years until that fateful day at forty-two. Once a woman realizes she's in the chrysalis of change, there's no turning back. The ground is shaky because our old self is slipping away, and we haven't yet learned who our new self is. That's one of the most complex parts of this journey: being in the gap, the chrysalis, with the high level of discomfort that seems never-ending. Thankfully, it doesn't last.

1.2 PERIMENOPAUSE: THE PRELUDE TO CHANGE

The landscape of a woman's reproductive life is rich and varied, with perimenopause being the "opening act" marking the beginning phase of transition. Often misunderstood and overlooked, this period sets the stage for menopause, unfolding in subtle yet profound shifts. In the prelude to change, it is here that the first whispers of transformation begin to echo. One of the fertility hormones, progesterone, begins a slow, imperceptible decline before estrogen's more dramatic shifts some period later.

Early Signs and Symptoms

For many women, perimenopause arrives unannounced, its presence signaled through a constellation of signs that hint at the shifts taking place. Menstrual patterns begin to fluctuate, with cycles that may lengthen or shorten and periods that can vary in intensity. Sleep may become less reliable, with restlessness and night sweats interrupting deep slumber. Mood swings, akin to those experienced in earlier hormonal fluctuations, may re-emerge, painting emotions in broad, unpredictable strokes. Most of it may seem like more extreme PMS, and like all the other months, we assume it will end soon, so we don't do much about it.

This initial phase can catch many people off guard, as these signs often blend into the fabric of daily life and are attributed to stress, lifestyle, or simply aging. However, recognizing them as harbingers of perimenopause allows for a proactive approach to managing what lies ahead.

Duration and Variability

The timeline of perimenopause is as individual as the women it affects. For some, this phase unfolds over a few short years; for others, it can span a decade, beginning in the early or mid-thirties. Such variability can make it challenging to pinpoint precisely when perimenopause begins and when it seamlessly transitions into menopause.

This variability isn't limited to duration alone. Symptoms can range from mild to severe, with some women experiencing a smooth transition with minimal discomfort while others navigate a more turbulent passage. This wide range of experiences under-scores the need for a personalized approach to managing perimenopause, which acknowledges its unpredictable and individualized nature.

Managing Symptoms

Navigating the early symptoms of perimenopause calls for a blend of strategies tailored to each individual's experience. Lifestyle adjustments almost always serve as the first line of defense. Simple changes, such as incorporating regular exercise into one's routine, can alleviate symptoms like mood swings and sleep disturbances. Nutrition also plays a pivotal role, focusing on whole and real foods rich in calcium and vitamin D to support bone health and phytoestrogens to potentially ease hormonal fluctuations.

Mindfulness practices, including meditation and yoga, offer another support layer, helping to manage stress and cultivate a sense of calm. The earlier a woman begins these practices, the better she engages them more easily, making the next phase as graceful as possible.

Preparing for What's Next

Perimenopause is not just a period of managing symptoms but also an opportunity to lay the groundwork for the years that follow. Prioritizing health and well-being during this time can ease the transition into menopause, setting the stage for a phase marked by vitality and resilience.

This preparation involves more than physical health; it's about nurturing well-being in its fullest sense. It means cultivating supportive relationships, giving yourself permission to prioritize your well-being, engaging in activities that bring joy and fulfillment, and creating spaces for rest and rejuvenation. It's about making informed choices regarding health care, staying proactive about screenings and preventive measures, and staying attuned to the body's signals. This period is for building the muscle of self-care so it's not overwhelming during the "main event." It's about taking your self-care game up a notch.

Equally, it's an opportunity to reflect on personal and professional goals, to practice trusting our choice to change rather than staying stuck due to fear, and to reassess and realign with what truly matters. For some, this may mean embracing new challenges or rediscovering passions long set aside. For others, it could involve slowing down and adopting a more measured pace of life that allows for reflection and connection. I have observed in the Western world that slowing down and practicing a more measured pace of life is an impactful medicine.

In essence, perimenopause invites a holistic approach to health that embraces the physical, emotional, and spiritual dimensions of well-being. By recognizing and responding to the early signs of this transition, women can navigate perimenopause with awareness and agency, making choices that successfully support their journey through menopause and beyond.

As this phase unfolds, it becomes clear that perimenopause is not just a prelude to change but a transformative period in its own right. It offers a window into the body's remarkable capacity for adaptation, a glimpse of the resilience that characterizes the female experience, and time to make small changes that add up to considerable support. In acknowledging and embracing this transition, women can move forward confidently, prepared for what lies ahead, and empowered to shape their journey through menopause and into the following years.

If any one woman has done this—and there have been many—you can, too. Reminding yourself of this may be helpful, especially during the more challenging moments. Another good reminder is that no hard pocket will last forever; in fact, it's a portal to something better.

1.3 THE MENOPAUSAL MILESTONE: SYMPTOMS AND SIGNALS

Menopause is defined as a point in time twelve months after a woman's last period. It's the "pause" of the menarche or the onset of the menstrual cycle. This milestone, while straightforward in definition, is anything but simple in experience. It's a time marked by significant shifts within the body, and each woman navigates these changes with varying degrees of intensity and symptoms.

Defining Menopause

Understanding menopause begins with recognizing it as a natural biological process, not a disorder or disease. It's a significant marker in a woman's life, indicating the end of her reproductive years and the beginning of a new phase. We tend to remember the ending part and forget the beginning part. It's always both. This transition, while natural, brings a host of symptoms that can affect a woman's quality of life.

Common Symptoms

The symptoms of menopause are as varied as they are common, impacting nearly every system in the body. Hot flashes often stand at the forefront of menopausal symptoms, characterized by sudden feelings of warmth, usually most intense over the face, neck, and chest, which can lead to sweating and even chills, day, or night. Sleep disturbances follow closely, with many women experiencing insomnia or waking frequently during the night. Changes in metabolism and weight gain can be particularly frustrating.

Changes in libido, mood swings, and vaginal dryness also present significant challenges, affecting relationships and personal well-being.

The physical manifestations of menopause extend into more chronic conditions as well. Osteoporosis becomes a concern due to decreased estrogen levels, which help maintain bone density. Similarly, the risk of cardiovascular disease can increase, making heart health a priority for menopausal women. Brain health also comes into play at this point, with many suffering from loss of memory and brain fog.

Navigating these symptoms requires a holistic approach, one that addresses not just the physical changes but the emotional and spiritual upheaval that can accompany this transition. It's about finding balance and seeking solutions that provide relief while nurturing the mind and spirit. I said it earlier, and I'll repeat it—the first step seems to be giving yourself permission to explore, experiment, and pursue a level of self-care that may be a whole new league for you. The key word is "permission." It's important, and only you can give it to yourself, so please do that.

Unique Experiences

What's crucial to understand is that no two women will experience menopause in the same way. Genetics, lifestyle, diet, and overall health play a role. Some women may breeze through menopause with minimal discomfort, while others find their symptoms nearly debilitating.

This variability can sometimes lead to feelings of isolation, confusion, and a sense of losing oneself. A woman may wonder why her experience differs significantly from her friends or other women in her family. Recognizing the diversity in experiences is entirely normal and underscores the need for personalized care and support.

Seeking Support

The significance of seeking support through this transition cannot be overstated. While it may seem harder to seek support if you feel overwhelmed and/or lost, finding your resonant support is vital. Open conversations with healthcare providers are crucial. Healthcare providers can offer insight into the range of treatments available, from natural hormone replacement therapy to alternative remedies, helping to tailor a plan that addresses your specific needs and concerns. If you open a conversation with a healthcare provider and are met with resistance, try again with greater clarity, or find another provider. You deserve to be supported.

Equally important is the support garnered from friends and family. Sharing experiences and strategies can provide practical advice and foster a sense of community, reducing feelings of isolation. For many women, support groups, whether in-person or online, become an invaluable resource, offering a space for connection, and understanding among those navigating similar changes. Try to find support that leans into solutions rather than getting lost in misery.

I was very open with my friends and family, and I found that it helped them understand and support me, as well as keeping me from feeling lost in shame and isolation. For me, the shame wanted me to believe that because I wasn't my usual capable self, I must be unworthy and no longer a viable member of society. As I worked through that, I realized it was a culturally programmed belief, and I could choose not to own that belief. That choice liberated me to embrace my journey without shame while cultivating a different version of myself as capable and viable.

Menopause marks a significant point in a woman's life with its myriad expressions and challenges. Yet, navigating this transition with resilience and strength through open eyes, understanding, support, and personalized care is possible. And it doesn't end once you cross the "twelve months with no menstrual cycle" finish line. You get to keep navigating and cultivating yourself as you learn and discover.

1.4 HORMONES AND HARMONY: UNDERSTANDING THE BIOLOGICAL SYMPHONY

In women's health, hormones play a lead role in a complex biological symphony that orchestrates everything from reproductive functions, glucose balance, thyroid function, and mood regulation, together referred to as the endocrine system. As we navigate through menopause, the fluctuations in hormone levels can sometimes feel like a discordant note, disrupting the harmony we've come to know. Within this adjustment period, understanding the role of hormones becomes crucial, not just for managing symptoms but for fostering a deeper connection with our bodies.

The Role of Hormones

Hormones, the body's chemical messengers, facilitate communication between different parts of the body. Hormones are essential to life and balance. There are many hormones—some of which you may recognize—like insulin, melatonin, Vitamin D (a hormone, not a vitamin), and cortisol. Estrogen and progesterone, in particular, have been the conductors of our reproductive systems, guiding us through menstrual cycles and pregnancies. These two hormones act as a natural check and balance system and usually do their jobs well during the fertile years. Of course, there is an increasing number of women for whom that's not the case, as with estrogen dominance, PCOS, and infertility, to name a few. As menopause approaches, the production of these hormones wanes, leading to a cascade of changes.

We'll address Hormone Replacement Therapy (HRT) or Menopause Hormone Therapy (MHT) in Chapters 2 and 4.

Achieving Balance

Restoring harmony amid hormonal fluctuations requires a multifaceted approach. Nutrition plays a foundational role; consuming a diet rich in phytoestrogens, omega-3 fatty acids, and vital minerals can support hormonal health. Foods such as flaxseeds, legumes, leafy greens, and fatty fish like salmon can be instrumental in this balance. Nutrition can be confusing for many women because there is so much contradictory information; until you can work with someone for an individual approach, I recommend you stick as close to the Mediterranean diet as possible because the research supporting it is the most far-reaching, consistent, and long-term. Then, you can adjust according to your needs.

Exercise and movement, too, emerge as powerful tools, not only for their well-documented benefits to physical health but also for their ability to modulate hormone levels, improve mood, and enhance overall well-being. I'm a proponent of cardiovascular exercise (e.g., walking, swimming, etc.), strength training (e.g., body weight exercise, weights, etc.), and stretching. Cardio, strength, and stretching form a powerful trio of balance, endurance, flexibility, and hormone stability.

Stress management emerges as another pillar in achieving hormonal harmony. Practices like yoga, mindfulness, meditation, creativity, and deep-breathing exercises can mitigate the impact of stress on the body, helping to stabilize hormonal fluctuations. For some, cultivating life force through practices such as Qi Gong or Tai Chi, which focus on harnessing the body's energy, can be particularly beneficial.

In the West, the cultivation and management of Life Force can seem foreign. Yet it is a foundational piece to not just graceful menopause but overall health and well-being.

For women who find lifestyle changes alone are not enough, judicious use of bio-identical hormones (BHRT) and, if necessary, medication may provide relief. It's essential, however, to approach this path cautiously, seeking guidance from healthcare providers well-versed in menopausal health.

Listening to Your Body

Tuning into the body's signals allows for a proactive approach to managing menopause. This act of listening goes beyond merely noting symptoms; it involves a deeper level of engagement with our bodies, recognizing the subtle cues and changes that may indicate imbalances. This may be new or familiar to you; either way, a deeper level of embodiment and listening is called for, which necessitates releasing fear and criticism of our bodies.

Embodiment practices, such as mindful movement or somatic experience, can enhance this connection. Virtually any movement, while present and embodied, will serve as a guidance system through the fluctuations of menopause.

Cultivating a Relationship with Your Life Force

Every particle of life in the Universe is a particle of light. Your body is made up of particles of light that become molecules, atoms, and cells that, in turn, create organs, glands, muscles, and bones.

It's all light. Light is Life Force, and Life Force is light. Most of us don't learn to directly relate to this energy. I encourage you to start now because it's personal medicine for you that costs nothing but your attention. Please see the resource information at the back of the book for instructions on how to do this.

Moving through Healthcare

Advocating for oneself in healthcare settings becomes an extension of this attunement. Equipped with understanding one's body and symptoms, discussions with healthcare providers can become more fruitful, leading to personalized care plans that genuinely resonate with one's needs and preferences. I realize this may be a scary proposition for some, yet for many women, this advocating for oneself (even in the face of a doctor and a large medical system) may be an aspect of growing their courage, confidence, and sense of empowerment.

A Holistic Approach

Embracing menopause with a holistic perspective acknowledges that the experience encompasses far more than physical symptoms —it touches every aspect of our being. Holistic means "whole," and we are coded for wholeness; this part of life is a call to that wholeness. Thus, managing menopause effectively calls for an approach that addresses not just the body but the mind and spirit as well.

- Physical Well-Being: Beyond diet and exercise, this includes adequate sleep, hydration, and addressing specific symptoms with targeted strategies, be it through conventional medicine, alternative therapies, or a combination of both.
- Emotional Well-Being: Acknowledging and addressing the emotional upheavals accompanying menopause is vital.

This may involve seeking support from friends, family, or professionals, engaging in activities that bring joy, and practicing self-compassion.

- Spiritual Connection: For many, menopause can be a time of spiritual reflection and maturation. Engaging in practices that foster a sense of connection to something greater than oneself—meditation, nature, a spiritual path, creativity, or religion—can offer solace and strength.

This holistic approach does not suggest a one-size-fits-all solution but underscores the importance of a personalized approach. It's about crafting a symphony of practices that resonate with each individual and that support health and well-being through menopause and beyond. You're creating a recipe with ingredients that come together for a balanced and pleasing outcome, and some ingredients may need to be modified along the way, which is okay and even uplifting.

As we navigate the complexities of menopause, understanding the interplay of hormones within our bodies and embracing a holistic perspective—one that honors the physical, emotional, and spiritual aspects of our being—we can move through this transition with grace and resilience, finding balance amid the fluctuations and embracing the profound awakening that menopause brings.

I remember reading a book on menopause during this phase, and the author said it could be another three to eight years. I almost threw the book across the room, thinking, "I can't do this for another three to eight years!" She wasn't wrong, but I was. It turned out that I did do it for another eight years while learning how to soften the resistance and create a recipe for better and better balance.

If you're wondering how the heck you're going to manage all these pieces, let alone fit them into your life, we'll address that in the coming chapters, so try not to worry too much as we're laying the groundwork. Besides, you have the rest of your life to practice.

1.5 POSTMENOPAUSAL: THE JOURNEY CONTINUES

With the winding down of menopause, a woman enters the postmenopausal phase, marking not an end but a continuation of her evolving narrative. This period often brings a newfound stability as the fluctuations in hormone levels that characterize menopause settle into a new normal. It's a time when the echoes of menopausal symptoms begin to fade, offering a clearer view of the path ahead—a path that, while filled with its own set of trials, is also ripe with opportunities for growth, vibrant health, and fulfillment.

Life after Menopause

The cessation of menopause symptoms ushers in a phase where women can redirect their focus from managing symptoms to optimizing health and well-being. Freed from the unpredictability of hormonal fluctuations, many find they can approach their health objectives with renewed energy and clarity. This period is an invitation to recalibrate, take stock of personal health and lifestyle choices, and make adjustments that resonate with their current needs and aspirations. It's a time for reflection and action—exploring new activities, hobbies, career direction, relationships, and passions that enrich life and contribute to a vibrant sense of well-being.

Long-Term Health Considerations

During post menopause, the landscape of women's health shifts, bringing certain conditions into sharper focus. Osteoporosis, for example, becomes a more pressing concern due to the decline in estrogen, which plays a crucial role in maintaining bone density. The risk of cardiovascular disease also increases, underscoring the importance of heart-healthy habits. It's essential to stay proactive about health screenings and preventive care. Regular check-ups, bone density tests, and blood pressure and cholesterol monitoring become key components of postmenopausal health care. A woman can effectively manage these risks by staying vigilant and working closely with healthcare providers, ensuring a more robust, healthier future.

- Bone Health: Incorporating weight-bearing exercises, ensuring adequate magnesium for calcium absorption, maintaining vitamin D intake, and following other recommendations from your healthcare provider.
- Cardiovascular Health: Prioritizing a diet rich in fruits, vegetables, and whole grains, healthy fats, lean proteins, maintaining a regular exercise routine that you enjoy, and managing stress effectively. A healthy heart also requires tending to past heartbreak, grief, and loss and making peace with how our lives unfolded. We may need to accept, forgive, and lovingly release certain aspects of our lives.

Maintaining Health and Vitality

Maintaining health and vitality in the postmenopausal years also requires a holistic approach, encompassing physical, emotional, and sexual well-being. Regular physical activity remains a cornerstone of health, with benefits that extend from improving cardiovascular health to enhancing mood and cognitive function. Nutrition continues to play a critical role, focusing on nutrient-dense foods that support deep cellular nutrition and energy levels.

Sexual well-being also deserves attention during this period. While some may experience changes in libido or vaginal dryness, these issues can often be managed successfully, allowing for a fulfilling sexual life if desired.

A New Beginning

Even if you are still raising children or caring for aging parents, the postmenopausal phase represents a new beginning—a chapter brimming with the promise of personal growth and exploration. Post menopause spans the remainder of one's life, often marked by a newfound self-awareness and a clearer vision for her future as a woman emerges from the challenges of menopause. This period offers the freedom to pursue interests and activities that may have been sidelined during earlier phases of life, whether that's traveling, taking up new hobbies, spiritual development, or even embarking on new career paths.

It's also a time for giving back, sharing wisdom and experiences with younger generations, and building connections that enrich both the giver and the receiver. Many find fulfillment in mentoring, volunteering, or engaging in community projects, leveraging their skills and experiences in meaningful ways.

This stage of life is characterized by a sense of liberation—freedom from the expectations and roles that may have defined earlier years. It's an invitation to live authentically, embrace the richness of life with all its possibilities, and step into a future defined by personal fulfillment, health, and happiness.

I used to share an office suite with a non-profit organization that supports women in third-world countries. Many of the volunteers for this organization were older, retired women, which I thought nothing of until I hit the peak of my own menopausal misery. I remember grabbing the arms of several women and desperately asking them if there was light at the end of the tunnel. Every woman said, "Not only is there light, but it's even better than before." These women were inches from me, and I could feel their truth. I tell you, I held on to their words like a lifeline. I can say they were right, including the part about "even better than before."

In the book *The Female Brain* by Dr. Louann Brizendine, she describes that a new brain tract comes online and gets laid during this phase of a woman's life, one that aids in living authentically by choice. I have found that as I discern and choose, it strengthens this brain tract, which then seems to improve my ability to be discerning and authentic. Saying "no" when I mean "no" and "yes" when I mean "yes" becomes easier and more natural, without the debilitating worry of how I'll be perceived that accompanies the younger years.

In this light, the postmenopausal phase emerges not as a period of decline but as a stage of life brimming with potential. It's a time to celebrate the journey thus far and anticipate the adventures ahead. With a focus on health, wholeness (however imperfect), and well-being, the postmenopausal years can be some of the most rewarding and vibrant of a woman's life.

"Menopause is not the end; it's a new beginning. Embrace the changes, and you'll find the strength within."

— ANONYMOUS

CHAPTER 2

UNVEILING THE TRUTHS OF MENOPAUSE

Imagine standing at the edge of a forest, the path ahead obscured by fog and the stories of those who've trodden before you, echoing with tales of beasts and brambles. This is how menopause often appears—a journey shrouded in myths and misconceptions, making it seem more daunting than it needs to be. Yet, with each step forward, guided by the light of knowledge, the path becomes more apparent, revealing not a treacherous trek but an enlightening passage. In this chapter, we spotlight some of the most common myths surrounding menopause, dismantling them with facts and empowering you with information to confidently navigate this transition.

2.1 MYTH VERSUS REALITY: WHAT MENOPAUSE IS NOT

Myth-Busting

- Menopause means aging: One prevalent myth equates menopause with aging, casting a shadow over this natural transition. While it's true that menopause marks the end of reproductive years, and it obviously happens around midlife, it doesn't spell the decline of vitality or beauty. Think of menopause as a seasoned tree in autumn, not withering but transforming, its colors more vibrant than ever. The silver strands in your hair or the laugh lines around your eyes are not just signs of aging; they're emblems of wisdom, resilience, and a life well-lived. You get to choose the qualities of this new and thriving identity, not based on culture but on how you rebirth yourself.

- Menopause ends your sex life: Another myth suggests that menopause puts an end to sexual desire and enjoyment, which couldn't be further from the truth. While hormonal changes can affect libido and comfort, they don't dictate the end of intimacy. With open communication, exploration of new types of pleasure, and sometimes a bit of creativity, menopause can herald a rich, fulfilling chapter of your sexual story.

Factual Information

Dispelling these myths requires a foundation of accurate information. For instance, while menopause does signify a change in hormone production, it doesn't halt the production of all hormones entirely. The body continues to produce estrogen, albeit in smaller quantities, through other tissues. This nuanced understanding can shift how we perceive menopause from an abrupt halt to a gradual transition.

The Impact of Misinformation

Believing myths about menopause can have tangible effects on mental health and self-perception. When menopause is viewed solely through a lens of loss, it can foster feelings of inadequacy or invisibility. Yet, when approached with facts and a positive outlook, menopause can be seen as a period of liberation and empowerment. Shifting the narrative around menopause helps lift the veil of stigma and fear, allowing women to approach this phase with optimism and openness.

I remember feeling a sense of losing myself as my "fertile self" seemed to drain away; then I realized my "fertile self" was only one aspect of my whole self. As I educated myself about this life stage, I realized that I was undergoing a rebirth, with the power to choose my direction based on the call of my soul. Embracing a unique version of beauty and evolving into the person I desired became possible, all nourished by the wisdom of a life well-lived and stewarded by grace.

Empowerment through Education

Educating ourselves about menopause is a powerful tool for changing the narrative. When women understand the physiological changes in their bodies, they can make informed decisions about their health and well-being. It also becomes easier to help those caring about us understand and be more supportive. Education fosters a sense of community, as sharing knowledge and experiences can help others feel less alone.

This chapter aims to empower women with knowledge, encouraging them to navigate menopause confidently and optimistically.

2.2 THE HORMONE REPLACEMENT THERAPY DEBATE: FACTS TO OVERCOME FEAR

Discussions on managing menopause frequently involve Hormone Replacement Therapy (HRT) or Menopause Hormone Therapy

(MHT). It's a treatment with polarized opinions, painting a picture fraught with controversy and confusion. Here, we aim to shed light on HRT, present the facts, and dispel fears to empower you with the knowledge to make choices that resonate with your health aims and lifestyle.

Understanding HRT

At its core, HRT involves the administration of hormones, typically estrogen, progesterone, and sometimes testosterone to alleviate the symptoms associated with decreased hormone levels during menopause. This decrease can lead to discomforts such as hot flashes, night sweats, mood swings, and a host of other symptoms that vary in intensity among women. HRT aims to bring hormones to levels that help manage these symptoms effectively, striving to bring a semblance of balance back to the body's hormonal ecosystem.

Weighing the Risks and Benefits

Recent studies have advanced our understanding of HRT, providing a nuanced view of its risks and benefits. It's crucial to recognize that HRT isn't a one-size-fits-all solution. For some, the benefits of symptom relief and potential protective effects for brain, bone, and heart health make it a compelling choice. For others, particularly those with a history of certain cancers, blood clots, or strokes, the risks may outweigh these benefits.

Research points toward an important timing factor in HRT's effectiveness and safety—the "window of opportunity" hypothesis suggests starting HRT closer to the onset of menopause may maximize benefits and minimize risks. This timing, coupled with the type of hormones used (estrogen plus progesterone) and the method of administration (oral, transdermal, or vaginal), significantly influences the risk-benefit profile of HRT.

The Women's Health Initiative (WHI) study in 2002 primarily focused on the effects of *synthetic* hormone replacement therapy (HRT), raising safety concerns. However, it's pivotal to understand that *bio-identical* hormones (BHRT), which have a structure identical to the hormones naturally produced by the body, present a different profile, potentially offering a safer alternative while still carrying a risk-benefit ratio for those seeking relief from menopausal symptoms. Unfortunately, there isn't as much research on BHRT because products that come from nature can't be patented and sold as widely as synthetically derived products; thus, less motivation for rigorous research. This is often where women slip through the cracks and encounter controversial viewpoints.

A healthcare provider may recommend a birth control pill or synthetic hormone replacement for women who have severe life-disrupting symptoms, and the allure to take them is often great. It makes no biological sense to take a birth control pill, which prevents ovulation, essentially giving your body the message of being pregnant when, in fact, your body is winding down fertility. It's a mixed message to the endocrine system when it's already in flux. I have found that more natural approaches, including bio-identical hormones, tend to be more balanced choices in the long run. Being offered only a birth control pill doesn't mean it's your only option; it just means you may have to research a little more and find a provider aligned with your wishes.

Personalized Medicine

The decision to pursue HRT should be as unique as your fingerprint—meticulously tailored to your health history, current symptoms, and overall wellness goals. A detailed discussion with a healthcare provider can illuminate the best path forward, considering personal risk factors and preferences. This conversation should delve into the duration of treatment, as recent guidelines suggest using the lowest effective dose for the shortest possible time to manage symptoms.

On the other hand, current guidelines may be overly conservative. Interestingly, nobody bats an eyelid when prescribing lifelong thyroid hormones for a low-functioning thyroid. Hormones decline as we age, just like enzymes and cannabidiols (yes, we have an endocannabinoid system just like we have an endocrine system). One must make decisions regarding hormones based on all the factors, including your personal comfort with how progressive or conservative to be.

There is limited research to support long-term BHRT use and limited research to support a shorter time. What's abundantly clear is that it is not recommended to stop and start multiple times. Take your time and make the decision that seems right for you.

Alternatives to HRT

For those who decide against HRT or for whom it's not recommended, a plethora of non-hormonal strategies can offer relief. These alternatives don't just stand in as backups; for many, they are preferred routes to symptom management.

- Lifestyle Adjustments: Simple tweaks in daily habits can significantly impact menopause symptoms. Staying active, maintaining a balanced diet rich in magnesium and vitamin D, and employing stress-reduction techniques such as yoga or meditation can all relieve symptoms.

- Phytoestrogens: Found in plants like legumes, flaxseed, and red clover, phytoestrogens mimic estrogen's effects on the body. Incorporating foods or supplements rich in phytoestrogens can help manage symptoms for some women.
- Non-Hormonal Medications: Certain antidepressants, blood pressure medications, and even anti-seizure drugs have shown efficacy in reducing menopause symptoms like hot flashes and mood swings. These options offer an alternative pathway for those seeking non-hormonal treatments yet may be a last resort for women who want a less pharmaceutical route.
- Acupuncture and Herbal Remedies: Acupuncture and herbal remedies hold promise for those inclined toward more natural approaches. Many women report symptom relief through these methods, highlighting the importance of a personalized approach to menopause management.

The dialogue around HRT, punctuated by advancements in research and evolving guidelines, underscores the importance of informed, individualized decision-making in managing menopause. With a clear understanding of HRT and BHRT's roles, risks, and benefits, alongside knowledge of alternative options, you stand empowered to navigate menopause in a way that aligns with your health and well-being aspirations.

2.3 BUSTING MYTHS ABOUT MENOPAUSE AND SEXUALITY

Amid menopause, the whispers about sexuality and its inevitable decline are both prevalent and misleading. In fact, this period can mark a renaissance of intimacy, unburdened by the concerns of contraception or the unpredictability of menstrual cycles.

Sexuality and Menopause

The narrative that menopause signals the end of sexual enjoyment is a myth that does a disservice to women everywhere. While hormonal changes can affect libido, they don't dictate the end of sexual activity or pleasure. Many find that this phase brings a newfound freedom and opportunity to explore their desires and sexuality in deeper, more intimate, and meaningful ways. It's a time for reinvention, where the focus shifts from procreation to pure pleasure and connection, both with oneself and with partners.

Maintaining Sexual Health

Navigating the changes in sexual health during menopause requires both knowledge and action. Here are several strategies that can maintain or even enhance sexual health and intimacy.

- Lubricants and Moisturizers: Vaginal dryness is a common issue that can hinder sexual enjoyment. Water-based lubricants and vaginal moisturizers can provide relief, making sexual activity more comfortable and pleasurable. Vaginal hormone cream is a consideration for vaginal dryness, which may contribute to a more enjoyable orgasm. It's okay to use both a vaginal hormone cream and a vaginal lubricant if necessary.
- Pelvic Floor Exercises: Strengthening the pelvic floor muscles through exercises like Kegels can improve sexual satisfaction by enhancing sensation and potentially increasing the intensity of orgasms.
- Mindful Sexuality: Approaching sex with mindfulness can deepen the connection with your partner, making intimacy more satisfying. It involves being fully present

during sexual activity, focusing on sensations and feelings rather than performance and outcome.

- Exploration and Communication: This period is an excellent time to explore new dimensions of your sexuality. Experimenting with different types of sexual activities and positions can add novelty and excitement to your sexual experiences.

Communication and Connection

Open and honest communication with your partner is critical to navigating the changes in sexuality during menopause. Discussing your needs, desires, and concerns can help both partners understand and adapt to these changes, fostering a deeper emotional connection and mutual satisfaction. Here are some tips for enhancing communication.

- Set aside Time: Dedicate time to talk about your relationship and sexual health without distractions. This can help both partners feel heard and valued.
- Be Open and Honest. Share your feelings, desires, and any challenges you're experiencing. Honesty builds trust and can lead to finding solutions together.
- Listen Actively: When your partner shares, listen actively without judgment. This can help you understand their perspective and build a more empathetic connection.
- Seek Support: Sometimes, talking to a counselor or therapist can provide the tools to improve communication and navigate changes in your relationship.

Seeking Help When Needed

For some, the changes in sexual health during menopause may require professional guidance. If you're experiencing sexual health issues that affect your quality of life, reaching out to a healthcare provider can provide relief and solutions. Seeking help is a proactive step toward maintaining your sexual health and ensuring your menopausal years are fulfilling and joyous.

Remember, menopause is not an ending but a new chapter in your life that brings changes and opportunities for expansion and exploration. By dispelling myths, embracing open communication, and seeking support when needed, you can continue to enjoy a healthy and satisfying sex life during menopause and beyond.

2.4 MENOPAUSE AND WEIGHT GAIN: SEPARATING FACTS FROM FICTION

The narrative around menopause often includes a chapter on weight gain, depicted as an inevitable part of the transition. This section aims to shed light on the reasons behind these body composition changes and offer strategies that support health and well-being without succumbing to the pressures of unrealistic body standards. It's time to shift the focus from the scale to a more holistic view of health.

Understanding Weight Gain

During menopause, the body undergoes a series of shifts, both hormonal and metabolic. As estrogen levels decrease, there's a tendency for the body to hold on to fat or adipose tissue, as it carries estrogen. This isn't just about aesthetics; it's a shift tied to biology. Moreover, our metabolism naturally changes as we age, compounding the challenge of maintaining the same weight or body composition as in younger years. The stress of menopause can increase cortisol, which tends to increase fat stores, particularly around the abdomen. These changes can feel sudden and frustrating, but they're rooted in the body's natural adaptation to this new phase of life.

- Hormonal Fluctuations: As estrogen declines, the body's way of processing starches and blood sugar alters, potentially slowing down metabolism and contributing to weight gain.
- Changing Metabolism: The natural aging process brings a gradual slowdown in metabolism, meaning a change of caloric intake is required as fewer calories are burned during rest and activity. I have found several things to counterbalance these changes:
- 1) High Intensity Interval Training (HIIT) twice per week
- 2) Intermittent fasting
- 3) Strength training twice weekly increases the caloric burn at rest
- 4) Only eat when hungry

I've had to train myself away from eating just because I want food and toward listening to my true hunger signals and following my body's lead. Of course, this is my recipe, learned through trial and error, and I encourage you to discover yours.

Managing Weight

Navigating weight changes during menopause doesn't demand drastic diets or rigorous exercise regimes. Instead, a balanced approach, focusing on nourishment and regular movement, can lead to sustainable health outcomes.

- Nutrition for Well-Being: Opt for a diet rich in whole foods, incorporating a diverse range of vegetables, fruits, lean proteins, and whole grains. These foods provide the nutrients your body needs to support its changing metabolism and help manage weight. Concentrated nutrition nourishes the cells at a deep enough level, so you don't have to "scavenge" for nutrients. Aside from emotional eating, not being nourished at a deep cellular level causes the feeling of not being satisfied or craving something, but you don't know what (aside from chocolate, which is on a throne of her own).

  ○ I prepare most of my food at home, so I know it's clean and real. Food not prepared at home tends to contain additives, which cause weight gain as the body strives to keep chemicals and toxins away from major organs.
  ○ I have learned these things to maintain a healthy weight through trial and error, and I encourage you to find the right recipe for you since we are all different.

- Regular, Enjoyable Movement: Finding forms of exercise you enjoy and can incorporate into your daily routine makes consistency easier. Whether walking, swimming, yoga, or dancing, regular physical activity helps boost your metabolism and enhances mood. Some women think that if they work out harder, they'll get the results they're looking for, but the opposite can be true. Any workout causes some inflammation; the harder the workout, the higher the inflammation, triggering a release of cortisol to lower the inflammation. This constant call on cortisol to release can potentially lead to weight gain and muscle injury. In midlife, the middle road is best. Not too much, and not too little.

- Mindful Eating: Pay attention to hunger and fullness cues, regulated by the hormones ghrelin and leptin. Eating mindfully can prevent overeating and help you enjoy meals more fully. Also, consider eating the rainbow, which is satisfying on many levels. When I'm cutting and eating colorful foods, my cells feel happy. It's a thing.
- Stress Management: Stress can lead to emotional eating and weight gain. Practices like meditation, deep breathing, or hobbies can reduce stress and its impact on your body. I believe stress management is one of the first key pieces to get good at because it will positively affect every other element of your journey in a helpful and peaceful way.

Self-Acceptance

Navigating menopause is as much about embracing the change as managing symptoms. Cultivating self-acceptance during this time is crucial. Your body is undergoing numerous transformations, and it's okay to acknowledge that it might not look the same as it did a decade ago. It's okay if some days are better than others. It's definitely OKAY if some days are a shit show. This isn't about giving up on health or fitness goals; it's about setting realistic expectations and treating your body with kindness and respect.

- Celebrate Your Body: Recognize all the incredible things your body does for you daily. Fostering gratitude for your body can shift your focus from criticism to appreciation.
- Use Positive Self-talk: Challenge negative thoughts about your body with positive communication. Remind yourself of your worth and beauty, independent of weight or body shape. Tips the scales in favor of acceptance and away from self-deprecation. Cells are intelligent and listen to

every word you say, they can only express your dominant narrative.

- Find Community: Connect with others going through similar experiences. Sharing and listening can be powerful tools for building self-acceptance and dismantling societal pressures around body image.
- Cultivate Creativity: Having a creative outlet—or several—can go a long way toward lowering stress, allowing you to express and accept yourself, and finding ways to settle into a new you.

Health Beyond the Scale

Finally, it's essential to remember that health extends far beyond what the scale reads. You are not a number but a mind, heart, body, and soul. Menopause is an opportunity to focus on holistic well-being.

- Comprehensive Health Checks: Regular health screenings become even more important during menopause. Monitoring blood pressure, cholesterol, bone density, and other markers can provide a clearer picture of your health than weight alone.
- Emotional and Mental Well-being: Pay attention to your mental health. Seek support when needed and engage in activities that bring you joy and fulfillment. It's important to discern between your mental experience of body changes and the things going on in your life that are mentally taxing. Each produces slightly different needs. Keeping a journal can be an excellent discovery tool and an outlet for maintaining your mental well-being.
- Quality of Life: Consider how your lifestyle choices impact your overall quality of life. Are you getting enough sleep?

Do you feel energized and engaged in your daily activities? These questions can guide you to make changes that enhance your well-being.

In this transition, when the body seems to be rewriting the rules, redefining what health and wholeness mean to you is an opportunity. It's about nurturing your body, mind, and spirit in ways that support you through menopause and beyond, focusing on well-being rather than numbers on a scale.

2.5 THE TRUTH ABOUT MENOPAUSE AND MENTAL HEALTH

Amid the physical changes, the emotional landscape undergoes its own transformation and is often overlooked in the broader discussion. The fluctuation of hormones doesn't just affect the body; it has a profound impact on the brain and mind, affecting everything from daily mood swings to more profound feelings of anxiety, lack of motivation, and depression. Recognizing and addressing these mental health challenges is as crucial as managing any physical symptom.

The dance of hormones during menopause, particularly the decrease in estrogen, is closely linked to mood. Estrogen interacts with chemicals in the brain that regulate mood, emotion, and cognitive function. As levels of this hormone decline, women may find themselves on an emotional rollercoaster, with feelings of sadness, worry, and irritability becoming more frequent visitors. One doesn't have to accept this as an unchangeable fact of menopause. Acknowledging the changes and doing your best not to resist them is the first step toward supporting yourself and finding strategies to significantly improve your mental well-being.

Actively reaching out for support is important for navigating these emotional waters. Talking to a healthcare provider can offer a starting point for managing symptoms, with therapy or counseling providing a space to explore feelings and develop coping strategies. But support doesn't only come from professionals. Connecting with friends, family, and especially others going through similar experiences can offer invaluable comfort and advice. There's strength in numbers; we find solace and practical ways to manage our well-being in sharing.

Several strategies have shown effectiveness in supporting mental health during this transition.

- Mindfulness and Meditation: These practices invite a moment of pause in our day, allowing us to observe our thoughts and feelings without judgment. Taking this pause will enable us to *sink* into our body, *soften* the tension, and connect to the *Source* of Life. This can help to manage stress and reduce feelings of anxiety or sadness. Remember... *sink, soften, Source,* so you can practice drawing into yourself alongside challenging feelings. You'll be amazed at how helpful this can be.
- Regular Physical Activity: Exercise releases endorphins, often called feel-good hormones, which can boost mood and overall well-being.
- Social Connection: Maintaining an active social life, even when challenging, can counter feelings of isolation and boost mood. Whether it's a coffee date, a walk with a friend, or a family gathering, these connections remind us of the joy in shared experiences.

The conversation around menopause and mental health is often silenced by stigma, leaving women to navigate these changes in silence. Breaking this silence and opening up about the emotional and psychological effects of menopause is crucial for change. It's in talking about menopause, in all its facets, that we dismantle outdated notions, replacing them with an understanding and acceptance that can transform this phase into a time of evolution and self-cultivation.

Recognizing the integral connection between body and mind paves the way for a transition marked by awareness and empowerment. The strategies and understanding we develop for managing mental health not only aid us through menopause but enrich our approach to life's challenges and transitions.

Every woman I know who has moved through menopause with grace has consciously and willingly let go of what no longer serves her in favor of what she's discovering does serve her—not perfectly, just consistently.

With this foundation, we step into the next chapter, ready to explore the holistic paths to well-being that menopause invites us to walk. In Chapter 5, we'll go into even more detail.

CHAPTER 3

NATURE'S PHARMACY FOR MENOPAUSE RELIEF

Imagine your kitchen, a place of nourishment and comfort, transforming into a healing sanctuary during menopause. The same natural wisdom that guides the growth of plants through the seasons can also support our bodies through this time of change. This chapter opens the door to the garden of natural supplements, a space where balance can be gently restored with the help of Earth's bounty. Here, we explore how integrating herbal allies into our daily routine can relieve symptoms, bringing us closer to harmony.

3.1 HERBAL ALLIES: NATURAL SUPPLEMENTS FOR SYMPTOM RELIEF

Nature offers a plethora of plants that have been used for centuries to ease the transition through menopause. Let's explore some of these herbal allies, backed by evidence, to understand how they can support us.

Herbal and Nutritional Supplements Overview

In the vastness of nature's pharmacy, certain herbs stand out for their ability to mitigate menopausal symptoms. Black cohosh, red clover, and sage make up a trio of powerful, natural allies. Each herb carries compounds that interact with our bodies in ways that can soothe and alleviate the discomforts brought by menopause.

- Black Cohosh: Black cohosh has been the subject of numerous studies, often hailed as a remedy for hot flashes and night sweats. Its roots whisper of centuries-old knowledge, offering relief and comfort.
- Red Clover: Rich in isoflavones, a type of phytoestrogen, red clover speaks to our bodies in a language similar to estrogen. It's particularly noted for its potential to ease hot flashes and improve bone health.
- Sage: Known for its cooling properties, sage can relieve fiery hot flashes. Its leaves, infused in tea or taken as a supplement, can also support mood and cognitive function. Mint might also do this for some women.
- Chinese Herbal Medicine: Imparts messages of intelligence through the five elements, life force or qi/chi, and the principles of yin/yang. Numerous options exist, recognizing that every human system is unique.

There are too many herbs to list here. Still, the key points are: 1) Consult a trained professional for personalized prescriptions, as online advice may not suit your needs, and 2) Primary care physicians generally don't specialize in herbal medicine, and it may not be realistic to expect them to have a broad range of understanding.

In working with hundreds of women over the years, I have observed that bringing a body back into balance naturally has a more lasting impact and fortifies the body in ways non-natural options can't.

Evidence-Based Benefits

The efficacy of these herbs isn't just folklore; it's grounded in research. Studies have shown that black cohosh can significantly reduce the frequency and intensity of hot flashes. Red clover, with its phytoestrogens, has been linked to improved bone density, while sage has demonstrated benefits in cognitive function and mood stabilization. While individual results may vary, the cumulative evidence supports these herbs as beneficial allies in managing menopausal symptoms.

Dosage and Safety Concerns

Navigating the world of herbal supplements requires understanding dosage and potential side effects. For instance, the recommended dosage for black cohosh often ranges from 20 to 80 mg per day, yet exceeding this amount or long-term use may lead to liver issues in rare cases. Red clover is generally considered safe but should be used cautiously by those with hormone-sensitive conditions. Sage, while beneficial, should be avoided in excessive amounts due to the presence of thujone, a compound with potential toxic effects at high doses.

- Always start with the lower end of the recommended dosage range.
- Monitor your body's response and adjust accordingly.
- Be mindful of any interactions with existing medications.

Consulting with Healthcare Providers

Before adding any herbal supplement to your regimen, you may want to talk with your health professional. They can offer personalized advice based on your health history and current medications, ensuring your foray into natural supplements is safe and effective. This dialogue also opens a broader conversation about integrating holistic approaches with conventional treatments and crafting a care plan that resonates with your unique needs.

Nature's pharmacy offers a treasure trove of remedies that can support us through menopause. By understanding the benefits and considerations of each herbal ally, we can make informed choices that enhance our well-being. Remember, these natural supplements are not just ingredients; they're messengers of healing, each with intelligence and potential to guide us toward balance and comfort during menopause.

3.2 DIET AND MENOPAUSE: FOODS THAT HEAL AND HARM

During the transformative phase of menopause, the body sends signals requesting different nutrients to support its new state. As estrogen levels ebb, the metabolic rate may slow, and the risk for certain health conditions can rise. Adjusting one's diet to meet these changing needs becomes a gentle act of self-care, providing the body with the resources to navigate this phase smoothly.

Befriending whole and real food is a revolutionary act during a time of assault on Mother Earth and her bounty. Consider that processed, chemical-laden food made in factories, not farms, is doing you no favors. In fact, food without a life force makes it harder for your body to find balance and produce energy.

Nutritional Needs during Menopause

The body's nutritional demands shift during menopause, spotlighting the importance of calcium for bone health, antioxidants for cellular repair, and fiber for digestive wellness. Incorporating a variety of nutrients helps counterbalance the hormonal changes, supporting overall health. It's also a time to focus on hydration, as water is crucial in maintaining cellular health, aiding digestion, and keeping skin supple.

Foods That Alleviate Symptoms

Certain foods have a reputation for easing menopausal discomfort, acting as natural soothers for the body's shifting landscape:

- Phytoestrogen-Rich Foods: Beans, flaxseeds, and sesame seeds contain phytoestrogens, which may mimic estrogen in the body, potentially easing hot flashes.
- Omega-3 Fatty Acids: Found in fish such as salmon and sardines, flaxseeds, and walnuts, omega-3s are known for their anti-inflammatory properties. They may help reduce the severity of night sweats and support mood regulation.
- Fiber: Whole grains, fruits, and vegetables provide vital nutrients, help maintain digestive health, and support a healthy weight.
- Magnesium to Increase Calcium Absorption and Vitamin D: Essential for bone health, magnesium—and for some women, calcium and vitamin D—can be found in dairy products, fortified foods, leafy greens, and fatty fish. These nutrients become increasingly essential to support bones as estrogen levels decline.

Foods to Avoid or Limit

Just as some foods can be allies during menopause, others may exacerbate symptoms, making it wise to consume them in moderation or avoid them altogether:

- Caffeine: While a morning cup of coffee is a cherished ritual for many, caffeine can trigger hot flashes and disrupt sleep patterns. Consider limiting intake or opting for decaffeinated beverages. I have found that the adrenal health of each woman is a good indicator of whether caffeine should be eliminated or just limited. If you drink coffee and feel "buzzy," it's too much for your adrenals. Another indicator is that if you take a week off coffee and have significant withdrawals, your system may be too sensitive to caffeine. If you notice no withdrawal symptoms and don't feel buzzy after a cup of caffeine, your adrenals may be in good enough shape to handle limited caffeine. Ideally in the morning to support your best sleep.
- Alcohol: Alcohol consumption can increase the frequency of hot flashes and contribute to weight gain. It can also affect sleep quality, so moderating intake is beneficial. My trick is to drink a glass of wine early in the evening and, ideally, take a walk afterward so the wine is metabolized before going to bed. If I don't do that, my sleep suffers. No more glass of wine with an 8:00 p.m. dinner, but hey, at least I can still have one with conscious timing!
- Spicy Foods: Some women may experience hot flashes when eating spicy foods, so observing how your body reacts and adjusting accordingly is useful.
- Processed Foods: High in salt, sugar, and unhealthy fats, processed foods can contribute to weight gain, affect heart

health, and lead to feeling lethargic. Brace for some news here. These foods should be eliminated. It is rough on a woman's body, already going through a stressful event, to handle sugar, unhealthy fats, and processed foods. It takes excessive life force or energy to protect the body from these foods, to break them down, and to eliminate them. The body often stores chemical-laden foods in fat tissue to sequester the toxicity away from organ function. And the body won't let go of the fat until there's a safe route out for the chemicals, inflammation, and toxicity. Detoxing off these foods is one of the best things you can do for your body.

Creating a Balanced, Menopause-Friendly Diet

Crafting a diet that supports your body through menopause doesn't have to be a complex puzzle. Focus on whole, nutrient-rich foods that provide a variety of benefits.

- Start with Color: Fill at least half your plate with colorful vegetables at each meal. This simple strategy ensures you get a wide range of vitamins, minerals, and antioxidants.
- Choose Whole Grains: Opt for whole grains like quinoa, oats, brown rice, and whole wheat, which provide fiber and help manage blood sugar levels.
- Include Lean Proteins: Incorporate lean proteins such as poultry, fish, and legumes to support muscle health and satisfy you.
- Healthy Fats are Your Friend: Avocados, nuts, seeds (flax being the queen), and olive oil offer healthy fats that support brain health and keep your skin looking its best.
- Enjoy Fruit: If your blood sugar is struggling, eat a maximum of two servings of fruit per day, ideally low-

sugar fruits such as berries. If your blood sugar is normal, up to three servings a day is okay.

- Stay Hydrated: Drink plenty of water throughout the day. Infusing water with fruits or herbs can make it more appealing and encourage you to drink more. Teas are also a healthy option.

There's no question that food prepared at home is healthiest, avoiding additives, extra sugar, and chemicals. Some women don't feel comfortable in the kitchen, and while some are willing to learn, others aren't. If you're not interested or able to prepare your own food, the next best thing is to use a meal delivery service that includes whole, real, and organic food delivered to you.

If you're willing to learn, in-person and online cooking schools exist. I took an online course to eat more plant-based meals and wanted good-tasting food. Start where you are and keep learning. I knew nothing when I began; little by little, I got better. I learned to make good soups, roasted vegetables, and many other things that keep me on track nutritionally, keep my weight stable, and save me a lot of time and money. Contrary to what most people think, preparing food at home does save time and money, especially when you cook in larger batches, which you can freeze or eat several meals from.

In addition to focusing on what to eat, consider how you eat. Enjoying meals slowly, savoring each bite, and being present with your food can improve digestion and meal satisfaction. It's also an opportunity to connect with loved ones, share meals, and create moments of joy around the table.

As your body transitions through menopause, listen to its cues, adapting your diet to meet its evolving needs. This isn't just about nutrition; it's about nurturing yourself, honoring your body's rhythms, and embracing the transformation with care and compassion. Through mindful choices and a heart full of deepening kindness toward yourself, navigating menopause can become a smoother, more graceful experience.

3.3 EXERCISE AS MEDICINE: MOVEMENT STRATEGIES FOR MENOPAUSAL WOMEN

In the dance of life, our bodies change rhythm as we approach menopause. It's a time when the music might seem too slow, but it's an invitation to find a new beat, a different way of moving that aligns with our evolving selves. In this context, exercise becomes not just a routine but a powerful ally, offering solace, strength, softening, and vitality. Let's explore how integrating movement into our lives during menopause can be transformative, profoundly supporting our well-being.

If you're already an exercise girl, please know that if some is good, more is not better. That tends to backfire during menopause when there's no extra repair capacity, leaving women with injuries, tendonitis, and pain that could all be avoided by finding your goldilocks zone. Not too much, not too little.

Benefits of Exercise during Menopause

The magic of movement unfolds in layers. On the surface, it helps us manage the physical symptoms of menopause, such as weight gain, moods, and hot flashes. Moreover, exercise strengthens our bones, combating the risk of osteoporosis, and enhances cardiovascular health, protecting our hearts as we transition through this phase. Above all, regular exercise cultivates a sense of well-being, grounding us in our bodies and reaffirming our strength and resilience.

Simply stated, all forms of life that don't move will deteriorate. A core tenet of Chinese Medicine is that qi, or life force, must move for there to be health. It's not a matter of "if" a human body should move; that's a given. Finding which kind of movement makes you happy is something you can be consistent with for the rest of your life. It's okay if that changes; just keep moving.

Tailored Exercise Recommendations

Finding the correct type of exercise that resonates with your body's needs during menopause is key. A blend of strength training, cardio, and flexibility exercises forms a holistic approach addressing the various health aspects impacted by menopause.

- Strength Training: Twice a week, engage in activities that build muscle mass, such as lifting weights, body weight exercises, or resistance bands. This boosts your metabolism and fortifies your bones, a crucial benefit as bone density tends to decrease after menopause.
- Cardiovascular Exercise: Aim for at least 150 minutes (i.e., thirty minutes five times weekly) of moderate aerobic activity each week. This could be brisk walking, cycling, rowing, or swimming. These activities support heart health and help manage weight, besides being excellent for uplifting your spirit. If you have enough energy, see if you can do High-Interval Intensity Training (HIIT) twice weekly in addition to moderate aerobic activity.
- Flexibility Exercises: Incorporate stretching, yoga, or Pilates into your routine to enhance flexibility, balance, core strength, and mind-body connection. These practices also offer the added benefit of stress relief, providing a calm harbor during hormonal tumult.

Overcoming Barriers to Exercise

Common obstacles can deter us from embracing physical activity during menopause, from lack of time to fatigue or even discomfort with changing bodies. Yet overcoming these barriers is possible with a few strategies.

- Schedule Your Workouts: Treat exercise like any other important appointment. Setting aside specific physical activity times makes you more likely to stick to your routine. I follow the principle of doing the most important things first in the day. Additionally, we have more energy earlier in the day; thus, prioritizing movement earlier in the day ensures it'll happen.
- Find Activities You Enjoy: The key to consistency is enjoyment. Whether it's a dance class, hiking, or gardening, choose activities that bring you joy and that you look forward to. If your body hurts, move in very gentle ways.
- Set Realistic Goals: Start with achievable goals to avoid feeling overwhelmed. Celebrate your progress, no matter how small, to stay motivated. Determine things like: 1) Do I prefer to exercise alone or with others? 2) Morning, afternoon, or evening? 3) At home, outdoors, or at a workout facility? 4) Can I keep a pair of walking shoes in the trunk of my car and use unexpected extra time by taking a walk? Ten minutes here and there adds up if taking a whole thirty minutes seems impossible. However slowly you start or need to go is better than nothing. Try not to compare what you can do now with what your younger self or anyone else could do.
- Seek Support: Joining a class or finding a workout buddy can provide encouragement and accountability. Sharing

the journey makes the process more enjoyable and less isolating.

Movement is a positive feedback loop—it feels good, so we naturally want more. If it doesn't feel good, it's worth discovering more about that. I've been moving daily for fifty-plus years. At least half of the time, I want to talk myself out of it. I give that voice a little airtime, and then the first thing I do is put my workout shoes on. Or fill my water bottle. Or set my weights up. That first step virtually guarantees I'll follow through even as I try to talk myself out of it. I also envision myself doing the exercise in my mind's eye, which is foolproof in drawing me into it.

At this point in my life, I work out independently and at home, except for walking and hiking. HIIT, weights, and stretching happen in the morning, with walking at night. Hiking is usually on a weekend day. I can't imagine all the extra steps of packing a gym bag, driving to a place, fussing before and after the workout, driving home, and unpacking the bag. I wouldn't stick to it. I've done it, and I know I don't like it. I'm too busy for it, but that's just me. If my life were less full, maybe I'd love the connection as much as the movement, but that's not the phase I'm in now. The point is to find your flow, do the things you enjoy consistently, and don't stop moving.

Starting Slowly and Building Up

If you're new to exercise or returning after a break, diving in too quickly can lead to burnout or injury. It's crucial to start slowly, allowing your body to adjust. Begin with shorter, less intense workout sessions and gradually increase the duration and intensity. This gentle approach honors your body's rhythms, making exercise a sustainable part of your life rather than a fleeting endeavor. Remember, the goal is not to reach peak performance overnight but to weave movement into the fabric of your daily life, creating a tapestry of health and vitality that supports you through menopause and beyond.

Movement fosters a deeper connection with our bodies, allowing us to live more embodied lives. Despite our culture emphasizing head-centric awareness, movement will cultivate a healthier relationship with your body, a vessel comprising 70 trillion cells, each holding a wealth of wisdom. Listen to your body to decide how, when, and what movements to engage in. A good motto is "feel" into it rather than trying to "figure" it all out.

3.4 SLEEP SOLUTIONS: RESTORING NIGHTTIME HARMONY

During menopause, one thread that often frays is our connection to peaceful sleep. This phase of life can turn the sanctuary of our beds into places where rest is elusive, and the night stretches long with wakefulness. Understanding how menopause influences our sleep and employing strategies to mend this thread can guide us back to restorative nights. I often hear, "I'm exhausted, so why don't I sleep?" I hear you; let's talk!

Impact of Menopause on Sleep

The shift in hormone levels that accompanies menopause directly impacts our sleep architecture, the structure that underpins a good night's rest. Falling estrogen levels are particularly disruptive, affecting our ability to fall asleep and stay asleep. They also make us more sensitive to environmental disturbances, like noise or light, further fragmenting our sleep. Our levels of melatonin, the hormone that regulates sleep cycles, change. Additionally, progesterone, known for its sedative and relaxation effects, decreases, stripping us of its sleep-promoting benefits. This hormonal upheaval paves the way for insomnia and can exacerbate sleep apnea in some women due to changes in the respiratory system.

Sleep Hygiene Tips for Menopausal Women

Creating an environment and routine conducive to sleep can significantly improve its quality. Make a clear decision that sleep is vital and that you'll tend to optimal sleep hygiene. Here are tailored strategies to rebuild our relationship with rest.

- Craft a Sleep-Inducing Environment: Keep your bedroom cool, dark, and quiet. Consider blackout curtains and white noise machines to block out disturbances. Ensure your mattress and pillows support a good night's sleep, inviting comfort rather than tossing and turning.
- Establish a Pre-Sleep Ritual: Develop a routine that signals to your body it's time to wind down. This might include reading, gentle stretching, or a warm bath. The key is consistency, as these cues help prepare your mind and body for sleep.
- Regulate Your Sleep Schedule: Strive for a regular bedtime and wake-up time, even on weekends. This regularity supports your body's circadian rhythm, the internal clock that dictates sleepiness and wakefulness.
- Mind Your Intake: Limit caffeine and alcohol, especially in the hours leading up to bedtime. Both can disrupt sleep patterns: caffeine delays sleep onset, and alcohol impairs sleep quality.
- Sleep Divorce: No one likes to talk about this, but you may not be able to sleep with your partner during menopause. If you're lucky enough to have an extra

bedroom with a comfortable bed, try it out for a few nights and see if you sleep better. At least have the option to move to a different bed if necessary. I now sleep in a separate room from my husband, and I know many women do. You may need to get support on how to broach this with your partner.

- Hormone replacement therapy: This tends to be an effective sleep solution for many women.
- CBD: Many women find CBD to be helpful for relaxation and even pain to optimize restful sleep.

Natural Sleep Aids

Incorporating natural remedies and practices can further support sleep, offering gentle, non-pharmacological options to encourage rest.

- Herbal Teas: Sipping on herbal teas such as chamomile, valerian root, ashwagandha, or lemon balm can be a soothing prelude to sleep. These herbs have properties that may relax the nervous system and promote sleepiness. I begin drinking relaxation teas in mid-afternoon to calm my system without drinking past 6:00 p.m., ensuring a better chance of not having to wake up to use the bathroom!
- Aromatherapy: Essential oils like lavender, bergamot, and sandalwood can be used in a diffuser or applied to pressure points. Their scents work through the olfactory system to reduce stress and induce calm.
- Supplements: Supplements such as melatonin and valerian might assist in keeping your sleep cycle more balanced and your system calmer. Dosage differs for everyone, so a little trial and error may be needed.

- Relaxation Techniques: Progressive muscle relaxation or guided imagery can be powerful tools. By focusing on relaxing the body part by part or visualizing a peaceful scene, you engage your mind in a way that can ease you into sleep and help you get back to sleep in the middle of the night.
- Mindfulness Practices: Mindfulness or meditation before bed helps quiet the mind, setting aside the day's worries and preparing for sleep. Even a few minutes can make a difference, creating a sense of peace that invites rest.

When to Seek Professional Help

While these strategies can be effective for many, there are times when professional guidance is necessary. If sleep disturbances persist despite your best efforts, impacting your daily life and well-being, reaching out to a healthcare provider is wise. Persistent insomnia, sleep apnea, or restless leg syndrome are conditions that not only disrupt sleep but can also have broader health implications. If it comes to this, a sleep specialist can offer a comprehensive evaluation, identifying underlying issues and developing a targeted treatment plan. This might include cognitive-behavioral therapy for insomnia (CBT-I), a highly effective approach that addresses the thoughts and behaviors that hinder sleep. They may also explore other interventions, ensuring your recovery to restful nights is grounded in understanding and tailored care.

Navigating sleep challenges during menopause calls for patience, understanding, and, sometimes, creative solutions. We can rekindle our relationship with sleep by tuning into our bodies' needs and adjusting our environment and routines. When needed, seeking professional help ensures we're supported in our quest for rest and guided by expertise and compassion. With these threads woven together, the tapestry of menopause can include nights filled with the deep, restorative sleep that fuels our days, allowing us to embrace this phase of life fully.

3.5 STRESS REDUCTION TECHNIQUES: MINDFULNESS, MEDITATION, AND MORE

In navigating the waters of menopause, the waves of stress can often seem higher and more challenging to sail through. Stress, a familiar companion to many, takes on a more potent form during menopause, exacerbating symptoms and impacting our well-being. Recognizing this, we turn toward ancient practices refined by modern understanding to anchor ourselves during these turbulent times.

The Role of Stress in Exacerbating Symptoms

The connection between stress and menopause symptoms is more than anecdotal; it's a well-documented phenomenon. Stress triggers the release of cortisol, a hormone that, in excess, can lead to a cascade of effects, including intensified hot flashes and disrupted sleep. It doesn't stop there—prolonged stress can touch every corner of our health, from heart health concerns to a dip in our immune system's efficacy.

I have thirty years of clinical observation that makes this connection explicit. A woman in any phase of menopause who has an increase in stress always experiences a worsening of her symptoms. Going through menopause is already stressful to the system; in general, life can be stressful, and added layers can put the system on tilt.

This is a compassionate reminder that our resistance to mind, body, and life changes is a huge stressor. The moment we release resistance, ease replaces the tension. The returns from this practice alone are in a class of their own.

Mindfulness and Meditation

As mentioned multiple times, mindfulness and meditation emerge as beacons of calm—they're practices that invite us to pause and find peace in the present moment. Mindfulness encourages us to engage fully with the present, fostering a heightened awareness of our thoughts, feelings, and bodily sensations without judgment. Meditation, often seen as a deeper dive into this conscious presence, offers a structured way to quiet the mind. Regular practice can lower stress levels, reduce symptoms of anxiety and depression, and even lead to lower blood pressure.

- Starting Small: Even a few minutes daily can make a significant difference. Apps and online guides can offer a gentle introduction to these practices. Almost everyone says they can't calm their mind, so they assume they're bad at it or doing it wrong. That is not true; everyone starts that way. It's a practice, and eventually, there is progress in settling the mind down; meanwhile, along the way, there are a gazillion other benefits to mindfulness and meditation in addition to settling stress. Even the Dalai Lama says some days he has a hard time quieting his mind, but he is consistent.
- Consistency is Key: Like any skill, the benefits of mindfulness and meditation grow with practice. Setting aside regular time each day fosters a habit that can change the whole landscape of your mental health.

Breathing Exercises and Yoga

Breathing exercises are simple yet powerful tools for navigating stress. Techniques such as diaphragmatic breathing or counting can help calm the nervous system, offering an immediate anchor in moments of stress. Yoga or tai chi, marrying breath with movement, extends this benefit with sequences designed to foster balance, flexibility, and inner calm. Yoga, with styles focused on relaxation and breathwork like hatha or yin, can be especially beneficial during menopause, addressing physical and emotional needs.

- Finding What Works for You: Exploring different breathing techniques and yoga styles can help you discover what resonates best with your needs. YouTube has videos for everything now—it's an excellent way to find some favorites before going to a live class to see if it's a fit.
- Incorporating Practice into Daily Life: Even outside of formal practice, mindful breathing can be a quick way to center yourself during the day.

Building a Personal Stress-Management Plan

Creating a personalized plan to manage stress involves weaving together various techniques that speak to your unique experience of menopause. Do this on paper or in a spreadsheet because if you leave it all in your head, it'll become a cloudy soup that may be hard to keep straight. It's about creating a toolkit that's as multifaceted as the symptoms and challenges you face. Here's how you can start.

- Assess Your Stressors: Identifying what triggers your stress explicitly can help you craft a more effective management plan. You can do this in one column on the left side of a page.
- Choose Your Techniques: Based on your lifestyle, preferences, and the nature of your stressors, select a mix of practices. This could include mindfulness, meditation, breathing exercises, yoga, or other activities that promote relaxation, such as walking in nature or engaging in a creative hobby. These could go in the right column of the page across from each stressor.
- Set Realistic Goals: Aim for small, achievable goals. This could mean starting with five minutes of meditation a day or one yoga class a week. Celebrating every baby step makes it more likely you'll continue.
- Reflect and Adjust: Regularly check in with yourself to assess how these practices are impacting your stress levels and menopause symptoms. Be open to adjusting your plan as needed.

In incorporating mindfulness, meditation, breathing exercises, and yoga into our lives, we not only weather the storms of menopause but also discover a deeper sense of calm and strength within ourselves. These practices invite us to slow down, breathe, and find moments of peace in a phase of life that often feels anything but peaceful. They remind us that amid the waves of change, there is an anchor within, a steady presence that we can return to again and again.

As we close this chapter on managing stress during menopause, we carry with us the understanding that the power to navigate this time with grace lies within our reach. We equip ourselves with tools through gentle discipline for this moment and life. It's a journey of discovering strength in softness, finding calm amid the chaos, and grounding ourselves in the present. With these practices in our toolkit, we step forward, ready to embrace the next chapter of our lives with open hearts and minds.

CHAPTER 4

HARMONIZING HORMONES: A PERSONALIZED PATH TO RELIEF

The stage is set, the lights dim, and in the quiet that follows, a single note pierces the silence—a clear, crisp sound that begins to weave a melody. This note, much like the decision to explore hormone therapy (HT) for menopause symptom management, marks the start of a new composition. The melody that follows can be as unique as the individual calling forth the music, a personalized harmony that seeks to balance the body's rhythm disrupted by menopause.

4.1 OVERVIEW OF HORMONE THERAPY OPTIONS

Hormone therapy, in its essence, is about restoring harmony. It's akin to tuning an instrument, ensuring each string vibrates at just the right frequency to produce a harmonious sound. For women facing the dissonance of menopause symptoms—be it the hot flashes that disrupt the day, the night sweats that mar restful sleep, or the mood swings that cloud mental clarity—HT offers a way to retune the body.

The options available in the realm of HT are diverse, each with its own set of considerations.

- Estrogen Therapy: The soloist in the world of HT, this option is often prescribed for those who have had a hysterectomy, delivering estrogen in various forms—pills, patches, drops, gels, and creams—to alleviate symptoms. Make sure to only take bioidentical estrogen and never alone.
- Progesterone Plus Estrogen Therapy: This duo works in concert to prevent endometrial cancer, which can result from estrogen alone, offering symptom relief while safeguarding health. ***Note: Bio-identical progesterone is the only choice I would make. Progestins are synthetic (meaning the molecular structure isn't the same as what our body produces). This is an important distinction (not all doctors agree), and I strongly agree with it. If you find an MD, physician's assistant, osteopath, or naturopath who will prescribe you progesterone, there is only one available, and it's called Prometrium. This is what to ask for.
- Take Both: It's essential to mimic the body's natural rhythms by taking bio-identical estrogen and progesterone together with or without a uterus. It's okay to take progesterone on its own (for example, in the early stages when you still have enough estrogen), but it's never okay to take estrogen HT alone. It should be estrogen together with progesterone, progesterone alone, or not at all.
- Low-Dose Vaginal Products: These localized treatments focus on specific symptoms, such as vaginal dryness or urinary issues, minimizing systemic effects.

Each option carries its melody, benefits and risks that must be considered in the broader context of an individual's health. The side effects, ranging from mild (bloating, mood swings) to severe (increased risk of blood clots or stroke), are the dissonant chords that must be weighed against the relief provided.

Individualizing Hormone Therapy

Tailoring HT is akin to composing a piece of music for a specific musician, considering their style, strengths, and their instrument nuances. This process involves:

- Understanding the Individual: This step involves thoroughly reviewing medical history, current symptoms, and lifestyle factors. It ensures that the therapy aligns with the individual's health landscape.
- Personal Preferences: Some may prefer the convenience of a patch over daily pills, while others might find topical applications better suited to their needs. These preferences play a crucial role in crafting a sustainable HT regimen.
- Risk Assessment: A qualified practitioner will recommend dosage and evaluate potential risks, such as a personal or family history of cancer, blood clots, or heart disease, to ensure the chosen therapy does not introduce unwelcome risks.

Monitoring and Adjusting Treatment

The journey with HT is not set in stone; it requires regular check-ins, akin to tuning an instrument before each performance. This monitoring process involves:

- Evaluating Effectiveness: Regular discussions about symptom relief and any side effects experienced help gauge the treatment's success.
- Adjustments: Based often on bloodwork and not often enough on feedback, the dosage or type of hormone therapy may be modified, seeking the perfect balance that offers relief while minimizing risks. Your feedback should be as important to adjustments as bloodwork, maybe even more important.

Each woman's menopause experience sings a different tune, one requiring a personalized approach to manage. From understanding the diverse options available and tailoring hormone therapy to fit individual needs to monitoring and adjusting treatment as necessary, the path to symptom relief is as unique as the individual journeying through menopause. Alternatives to traditional hormone therapy provide additional options, offering a chorus of possibilities for those seeking harmony amid change.

Elizabeth arrived in my office exhausted, withered, and dry; she had no motivation, wasn't sleeping, and cried all the time. I knew that appearance and feeling from my experience and the hundreds of women I've worked with. She wanted hormones, and within a week, she was sleeping, had energy again, her emotions stabilized, and, as a professor, she was back to herself again. The other exciting thing is she had moisture in her skin and was no longer withered-looking.

4.2 BEYOND HORMONES: OTHER MEDICAL OPTIONS FOR SYMPTOM MANAGEMENT

In the realm of menopause management, the path to relief is adorned with a variety of treatments beyond hormone therapy. It's a landscape where modern medicine meets age-old wisdom, offering options tailored to alleviate the multifaceted symptoms of menopause. This section explores the richness of this terrain, guiding you through non-hormonal prescription medications, interventional therapies, vaginal health treatments, and strategies for osteoporosis prevention and treatment. Each offers a beacon of hope, a way to navigate the changes your body is experiencing with dignity and comfort.

Non-Hormonal Prescription Medications

For those who seek solace from the disruption of menopause symptoms but find hormone therapy not to their liking or not suitable due to health reasons, non-hormonal prescription medications present a viable alternative. These medications, often repurposed from their original use, have been found to offer significant relief for specific symptoms:

- SSRIs and SNRIs: Originally developed for depression and anxiety, certain SSRIs (Selective Serotonin Reuptake Inhibitors) and SNRIs (Serotonin and Norepinephrine Reuptake Inhibitors) have proven effective in reducing hot flashes. Their role in mood stabilization also makes them a dual-purpose option for those navigating the emotional rollercoaster of menopause.
- Gabapentin: Known primarily as a treatment for seizures, gabapentin has shown promise in reducing hot flashes and improving sleep quality for menopausal women.
- Clonidine: Typically used to treat high blood pressure, clonidine can also help alleviate hot flashes, offering an alternative for those who may not be candidates for other treatments.

While effective, these medications have their own considerations. Side effects and interactions with other medications are factors to discuss with your healthcare provider to ensure the choice aligns with your overall health profile and menopause management goals.

Integrative Therapies

Beyond traditional medication, integrative therapies like acupuncture and chiropractic care offer a holistic approach to symptom management. Rooted in centuries of practice, these therapies provide relief by addressing the body's energy flow and structural alignment.

- Acupuncture: This ancient practice involves the insertion of thin needles at specific points on the body, aiming to restore balance and flow to the body's energy, regulate hormones, strengthen organ function, and lower stress. Many find acupuncture effective in reducing hot flashes, improving sleep, lowering stress, and enhancing overall well-being.
- Chiropractic and/or Osteopathic Care: Focusing on the body's structure, particularly the spine, adjustments can help alleviate menopause-related joint pain and improve nervous system function, contributing to overall symptom relief.

Incorporating these therapies into your menopause management plan can provide a complementary approach, addressing this transition's physical and emotional aspects.

Vaginal Health Treatments

Menopause can significantly affect vaginal health, leading to dryness, discomfort, and pain during intercourse. Thankfully, various treatments specifically address these concerns, offering relief and restoring comfort.

- Lubricants and Moisturizers: Over-the-counter options like water-based lubricants and vaginal moisturizers can provide immediate relief for dryness and discomfort, making sexual activity more enjoyable and reducing daily discomfort.
- Low-Dose Vaginal Estrogen: For those who need more than lubricants and moisturizers, low-dose vaginal estrogen products (available as creams, tablets, or rings) offer a localized treatment that minimizes systemic absorption, making it a safer option for many women.

These treatments, while effective for vaginal symptoms, should be chosen in consultation with a healthcare provider, ensuring they fit within your overall treatment plan and health considerations.

Osteoporosis Prevention and Treatment

The decrease in estrogen during menopause doesn't just affect temperature regulation and mood; it also impacts bone density, increasing the risk of osteoporosis. Addressing bone health is a critical component of menopause management, with strategies focusing on prevention and treatment.

- Magnesium and Vitamin D: A diet rich in magnesium assists calcium absorption, and it, along with vitamin D, supports bone health. Magnesium is depleted in soils which means levels are low in food. Most people don't get enough skin exposure without sunscreen which makes supplements highly recommended to reach the required daily intake for both.
- Exercise: Weight-bearing and muscle-strengthening exercises are pivotal in maintaining bone density and preventing osteoporosis.

Preventive measures, including regular bone density screenings, ensure that any loss is detected early, allowing for timely intervention.

Navigating menopause calls for a comprehensive approach that addresses the symptoms and the long-term health implications of this natural transition. From exploring non-hormonal medications and interventional therapies to prioritizing vaginal and cardiovascular health and bone density, the options available provide a rich array of solutions. Because each woman's experience with menopause is unique, so, too, should be her path to comfort and health during this phase of life.

4.3 THE ROLE OF SURGERY IN MENOPAUSE MANAGEMENT

Navigating through the waves of menopause, some women find themselves considering surgical options to address issues that arise during this period of change. It's a decision that brings many considerations, from the nature of the procedure to the recovery process and its implications on one's overall wellness during menopause.

When Surgery Is Considered

Surgery emerges as a path to relief in specific scenarios when other treatments have not provided adequate results. Conditions such as uterine fibroids, which can cause heavy bleeding, pain, and other symptoms, may necessitate surgical intervention. Similarly, endometrial ablation is a procedure often looked to for resolving heavy menstrual bleeding that doesn't respond to less invasive treatments. These decisions are deeply personal, hinging on various factors, including the severity of symptoms, the impact on daily life, and the potential for improvement through surgery.

- Uterine fibroid removal, known medically as myomectomy, can relieve symptoms like heavy bleeding and pelvic discomfort as a last resort.
- Endometrial ablation, aiming to reduce menstrual flow, may be suggested when bleeding is so severe that it disrupts daily activities.

Understanding Surgical Options

The landscape of surgical options is vast, each with its contours of risks and benefits. A myomectomy, for instance, offers relief from the symptoms of fibroids but with considerations such as the possibility of fibroids returning or complications during surgery.

- Hysterectomy: The complete removal of the uterus, a more definitive solution for fibroids, heavy bleeding, or other uterine issues, ends menstruation and the ability to conceive.

- Oophorectomy: The removal of one or both ovaries, often considered in cases where there's a high risk of ovarian cancer, drastically alters hormone levels and accelerates menopause symptoms if not already in perimenopause.

Each procedure has its benefits and should be considered following detailed discussions with healthcare providers about what to expect.

Recovery and Post-Surgical Care

The post-surgery period is a time of healing, both physical and emotional. Recovery can vary widely depending on the type of surgery and the individual, from managing pain and preventing infection to adjusting to changes in the body and its functions. Support from healthcare teams, family, and friends plays a crucial role in this process, providing the care and encouragement needed for a full recovery. It's a period where the body mends and adjusts, a time to nurture and strengthen the connection with the energetic hub of the womb.

- After a myomectomy, recovery might include managing pain and a gradual return to normal activities, with a focus on healing and monitoring for any signs of complications.
- Following endometrial ablation, one might experience changes in discharge and menstrual patterns as the body adjusts. It's a time for rest and monitoring, ensuring the desired outcome of the procedure is achieved.

Making an Informed Decision

The decision to pursue surgery is significant, requiring understanding the potential outcomes, risks, and benefits. It's a conversation that involves not just the individual considering surgery but also their healthcare providers, family, and support network.

- Gathering information about all available options, including less invasive treatments, provides a foundation for making an informed choice.
- Discussing potential outcomes, both desired and possible complications help set realistic expectations for what surgery can and cannot achieve.
- Considering the impact of surgery on menopause symptoms, hormone management, and overall health is crucial. For some, surgery may offer relief and a path to improved quality of life. For others, the risks may outweigh the benefits.

In the landscape of menopause management, surgery is a path that some may walk. It's a decision marked by careful consideration, informed by a deep understanding of the individual's health, needs, and the potential for improved quality of life. As with any aspect of menopause management, it's a choice that is deeply personal, reflecting not just the desire for relief but also the hope for a future marked by wellness and vitality.

4.4 CREATING A HEALTH CARE TEAM: FINDING THE RIGHT SUPPORT

Navigating menopause can often feel like trying to read a map without a compass; you know where you need to go, but the path is unclear. This is where building a dedicated healthcare team becomes invaluable, acting as your compass through this phase of life. The right team can provide medical support, guidance, understanding, and a holistic approach to your well-being.

Assembling a Multidisciplinary Team

Crafting a team that addresses the multifaceted aspects of menopause means looking beyond your general practitioner. This team might include:

- Gynecologists, physician's assistants, and naturopaths are specialists in women's reproductive health, offering insights into hormonal changes and managing menopause symptoms. Any other specialist (e.g., urologist) should be seen as needed.
- Nutritionists: Experts in diet and its effects on the body, they can help you adapt your nutritional intake to support your health during menopause.
- Chinese Medicine: Practitioners are well versed in the whole body, treating both the root cause and the symptom. Chinese medicine may include acupuncture, herbal formulas, nutrition, breathing exercises, energy or life force management, stress management, alchemical healing (soul-level healing), creative expression, or tapping.
- Physical Therapists: These professionals can recommend exercises to maintain bone density, improve sleep, and reduce stress.
- Mental Health Professionals: These therapists or counselors can support you through the emotional and psychological changes that accompany menopause.

Each professional brings a unique perspective, contributing to a comprehensive approach that addresses the physical symptoms and the emotional and mental health challenges that may arise.

The Importance of Communication

Open dialogue with your healthcare team is crucial. It ensures everyone is aligned with your health goals and understands your concerns and preferences. Tips for effective communication include:

- Be Open and Honest: Openly share your symptoms, fears, and lifestyle. The more your team knows, the better they can tailor their advice.
- Ask Questions: No question is too small. Understanding your health and treatment options empowers you to make informed decisions.
- Share Updates: Keep your team informed about any changes in your symptoms or concerns. This ongoing dialogue allows for adjustments in your care plan as needed.

Effective communication fosters a partnership between you and your healthcare team, ensuring you feel supported and understood. On the other hand, navigating a multidisciplinary team without a principal conductor or coach may seem confusing, sort of like a "who's on first" situation. If you don't feel capable of doing that, consider appointing a health advocate. While it may seem over the top, there's nothing wrong with starting a spreadsheet to keep track of who said what, recommendations made, what's working, etc.

Leveraging Community Resources

Beyond your direct healthcare team, numerous community resources can offer support and information:

- Support Groups: Connecting with others who are going through similar experiences can provide comfort, understanding, and practical advice.
- Educational Workshops: Many community centers and health clinics offer nutrition, exercise, and stress management workshops during menopause.
- Online Forums: Digital platforms can be a rich source of information and support, allowing you to access a wide range of experiences and advice.

These resources complement the advice from your healthcare team, providing a broader support network that can help you navigate menopause confidently.

Crafting your healthcare team for menopause is more than finding experts; it's about building a support system that encompasses all aspects of your well-being. From medical professionals to community resources, each element guides you through this change with care, understanding, and personalized attention.

4.5 PREPARING FOR YOUR MENOPAUSE CONSULTATION: QUESTIONS TO ASK

Walking into a doctor's office can often feel like stepping onto a stage without knowing your lines. The spotlight is on, but the words escape you. This sensation can be even more pronounced when the topic is as personal and complex as menopause. To ensure you make the most of your consultation, do a bit of preparation to turn apprehension into empowerment.

Getting Ready for Your Appointment

Gathering your thoughts and information is key before the curtain rises on your consultation. This preparatory step is like tuning your instrument before a performance, ensuring everything is set for a harmonious exchange.

- Symptom Journal: Keep a detailed record of your symptoms, noting their frequency, intensity, season, and any triggers you've observed. This diary becomes a valuable tool, offering your healthcare provider insights into your experience. The more concise you are, the more likely you'll be taken seriously. Be clear and straightforward, and it will help you get the best the doctor(s) have to offer.
- Medication and Supplement List: Compile a comprehensive list of all medications and supplements you're currently taking, including dosages. This information helps avoid potential interactions with any new treatments recommended.
- Personal Health History: Be ready to discuss your personal and family health history, mainly related to cancer, heart disease, and osteoporosis, as these can influence your treatment options.
- Visioning: If you're still nervous after preparation, visualize yourself remaining calm and composed during the appointment. Centering yourself in respect and dignity enhances the likelihood of receiving respectful treatment. Research indicates that replacing worry with a clear vision

multiple times before your appointment improves the odds in your favor.

Essential Questions to Pose

Armed with your symptom journal, health information, and dignity, you're now ready to engage in a meaningful dialogue with your healthcare provider. While medical treatments are often a focus of menopause management, lifestyle modifications and alternative treatments can play a pivotal role in alleviating symptoms. Crafting a list of questions in advance can guide this conversation, ensuring you cover all areas of concern.

- What are the most effective treatments for my specific symptoms?
- Are there any lifestyle changes you recommend that could help alleviate my menopause symptoms?
- How do my current health conditions affect my treatment options for menopause?
- Can you explain the risks and benefits of hormone therapy, considering my health history?
- What non-hormonal treatments are available, and how effective are they?
- Are there any alternative or complementary therapies that might benefit me?
- How will we monitor the effectiveness of my treatment plan and adjust if necessary?
- What stress management options would be good for me?
- Add to this list as you learn and discover more about yourself.
- Take notes during the appointment so details can be remembered.

Charting the Course for Follow-up and Ongoing Care

Menopause management is not a one-time event, but a dynamic process that unfolds over time. Setting the stage for ongoing care is crucial for adapting your treatment plan as your needs evolve.

- Ask about the frequency of follow-up appointments and what to expect during those visits.
- Discuss how you can communicate any changes in your symptoms or concerns between appointments.
- Inquire about any additional screenings or tests—such as blood work and breast or bone density scans—that may be needed to monitor your health in a comprehensive manner.

With these preparations and discussions, you can step confidently into your menopause consultation, ready to engage in an informed and productive dialogue with your healthcare provider. This proactive approach not only demystifies menopause but also places you at the center of your care, empowered to make decisions that best support your journey through this natural phase of life.

If you experience any of the following, it would be in your best interests to bring it up or move on to a more supportive practitioner:

- The feeling of not being listened to or heard
- Being rushed through your consultation
- Experiencing dismissal or belittlement of your symptoms
- If condescension is the tone of how you're being treated

Sure, practitioners are busy, but plenty of healthcare professionals can handle their schedules and your needs with warmth, honesty, and heart. Find them.

As we close this chapter, remember that menopause, with its myriad changes and challenges, also opens the door to growth at every level of your being. The conversations you have, the questions you ask, and the choices you make about your care are all steps on the path to understanding and embracing this phase of life. With the proper support and information, you can navigate menopause with confidence, finding strategies that resonate with your body and spirit. As we look ahead, let the insights gained here light the way, guiding you toward a future where menopause is not an ending but a new beginning, rich with possibilities for health and happiness.

CHANGING THE NARRATIVE
AROUND MENOPAUSE

"The trick is to age honestly and gracefully and make it look great so that everyone looks forward to it."

— *EMMA THOMPSON*

I told you at the beginning of our journey together that menopause is not just a transition but an awakening... but for some women, the thought of it is so terrifying that it's hard to even imagine it as a transition. It feels like more of an ending. This is largely due to how it's been viewed by society for such a long time.

We're trained to think of it as a mark of the end of our youth and vitality, but the reality is that youth doesn't end abruptly like this – it's a spectrum, one that we're transitioning along throughout our whole lives. Nothing ends when we hit menopause. It is simply a time of transformation and awakening the next phase of ourselves.

When we navigate menopause with knowledge and wisdom, it becomes an opportunity, and we unlock vitality we haven't felt in years. Hopefully, even if you were feeling less than enthusiastic about it when you picked up this book, by now you're beginning to see the hope and opportunity this phase of life has to offer, and it's with this in mind that I'd like to ask you to reach out a helping hand to other women approaching menopause.

That sounds like a lot, but all I need you to do is write a short review. Let me explain.

By leaving a review of this book on Amazon, you'll make sure that it's a positive and empowering view of menopause that

women find when they're looking for guidance about this phase of life.

Reviews shine a light on the information new readers are looking for, and they show them where they can find what they're looking for. By guiding women in the direction of this book, you'll not only help them prepare for what's ahead; you'll show them that menopause isn't the ending they fear: It's an opportunity for awakening.

Thank you so much for your support. Together, we can change the narrative.

Scan the QR code below

CHAPTER 5

EMBRACING EMOTIONAL EQUILIBRIUM

I magine standing in the eye of a storm, the world swirling around you in a frenzy of wind and rain. Yet, in this space, there's an unexpected calm, a center of stillness that holds firm despite the chaos. Menopause, with its emotional highs and lows, often feels like navigating through a cyclone. But within, there's a potential for equilibrium, a chance to find your calm center. This chapter is about tapping into that inner stillness, transforming the emotional rollercoaster of menopause into a journey of emotional balance and self-discovery.

5.1 MOOD SWINGS AND MORE: EMOTIONAL HEALTH DURING MENOPAUSE

The emotional landscape of menopause is as varied as the individuals experiencing it. Moments of joy and sudden irritation or sadness become part of the day's unpredictable weather. It's like the weather in spring, where sunshine quickly turns to rain, reflecting the swift changes in our emotional state during menopause.

The Emotional Roller Coaster

For many, this period is marked by mood swings that feel as though they come without warning. One minute, you might find laughter bubbling up from within, and the next, tears are inexplicably close to the surface. It's akin to watching a scene from your favorite comedy only to have it switch to a heart-wrenching drama without any notice. Noticing this without judgment and with compassion is your best medicine.

Biological Underpinnings

The root of these mood fluctuations often lies in the shifting sands of our hormonal landscape. Estrogen plays a crucial role in regulating mood by influencing the production and function of serotonin, a neurotransmitter that contributes to feelings of well-being and happiness. As estrogen levels ebb and flow, so too does our emotional stability, leaving us feeling like we're at the mercy of an unpredictable tide.

Strategies for Stability

Finding your equilibrium amid these shifts is key. Consider these approaches:

- Mindfulness Practices: Simple techniques, such as focusing on your breath, being *in* your body, or practicing gratitude, can anchor you in the present moment and offer a break from the storm of emotions.
- Regular Exercise: Physical activity is not just about keeping the body fit; it's a powerful mood stabilizer. A brisk walk, a cycle through the park, or any activity that

gets your heart pumping can lift your spirits and steady your mood.

- Professional Guidance: Sometimes, the emotional waves of menopause can feel overwhelming. Reaching out to a therapist or counselor provides a safe space to explore these feelings and develop coping strategies.

The Importance of Self-Compassion

During these turbulent times, being kind to yourself is essential. Self-compassion isn't about indulgence; it's about acknowledging your experience with kindness and understanding. Self-compassion is a powerful medicine. When emotions surge, remind yourself that this is a natural part of menopause, not a sign of weakness. Embrace self-care activities that resonate with you, whether taking a long bath, reading a book, or spending time in nature. Each act of self-kindness is a step toward emotional balance.

The part of us that may take a hit during menopause is our self-esteem and self-worth. Ample hormones during the fertile years can mask our insufficient self-compassion and self-acceptance. All the tools in this book are designed to support your self-acceptance, value, and, ultimately, your self-love. Let it be a compassionate process and permanent practice as you build the muscle of emotional strength.

Mood Tracking Chart

Consider keeping a mood-tracking chart to help you understand your emotional patterns. This simple tool can help you visualize the ebb and flow of your emotions, making it easier to identify triggers and find effective coping strategies. You can create your chart with columns for the time of day, the emotion experienced, potential triggers, and notes on how you navigated through it. Over time, this chart becomes a valuable resource for recognizing patterns and planning proactive steps for emotional well-being.

Reflective Journaling Prompts

Journaling offers a private, reflective space to process your emotions. Here are a few prompts to get you started.

- What emotion surprised me today, and how did I respond?
- When did I feel most balanced today, and what contributed to that feeling?
- How did I practice self-compassion today, and how did it make me feel?

Moving Emotions Creatively

Exploring creative ways to move your emotional energy can be potent. Anything you do that feels creative, done with intention, can move emotional energy within moments. The following are a few ideas to consider:

- Keep a sketchbook dedicated to your journey, using pages like an "altar" upon which you write, draw, paint, or collage your feelings on the left side and your preferences on the right. You intend to transform or "alter" emotional energy into relief, release, and more serving feeling states.
- Use watercolor pencils in a mixed-media journal to write a genuine letter about your struggles to yourself or the Universe. Then, take a brush, dip it in water (you may need to do this a few times), and blur the written words while holding your intention in your

heart. You can write new words or sentences or collage your chosen intention on top when it dries. This represents a dissolving of old energy in favor of new.

- Plant some flowers or herbs with the intention that Mother Earth receive your emotions and grow them into something beautiful.
- Choose clothing with colors that lift your spirit. Keep in mind that black is devoid of life force, and red tends to incite irritation. Supportive colors may be white, gold, blue, green, violet, and pink.
- Take an art class to simply play.
- Choose a particular uplifting color each day and see how many times you notice it. Let that color represent an intention.

5.2 BUILDING A SUPPORTIVE COMMUNITY: YOU ARE NOT ALONE

In the heart of the menopausal transition, where emotions can fluctuate as rapidly as a breaking wave, finding a harbor in the form of a supportive community becomes a comfort and a necessity. This network of friends, family, and peers can buoy us through the choppy waters, offering solace, understanding, and camaraderie.

Leveraging Online Resources

In today's digital age, the internet offers a vast expanse of forums, social media groups, and virtual meetups, each a potential thread in the web of your supportive community. Online platforms can dissolve geographical barriers, allowing you to connect with individuals from diverse backgrounds and perspectives. When seeking out these virtual spaces, look for groups that foster positive, supportive discussions and that respect privacy.

The Role of Community in Healing

The healing power of community during menopause cannot be understated. In sharing your story and listening to others, a mutual exchange of wisdom and comfort unfolds. This exchange, akin to the gentle give and take of the sea with the shore, can provide emotional solace and practical advice, enriching your menopausal experience. Maybe it's a girlfriend you walk with regularly or a larger group of women who share their stories. This sense of belonging can significantly mitigate feelings of isolation, reminding you that, though the journey might be deeply personal, you are not navigating it in solitude.

In fostering connections, you create a network of support that not only guides you through menopause but also enriches your life beyond it. This community becomes a testament to shared strength, a beacon for those still finding their way, and a reminder of the profound connections that sustain us through every season of life.

5.3 THE POWER OF STORYTELLING: SHARING YOUR MENOPAUSE EXPERIENCE

Every thread contributes to the story's richness in the tapestry of life. Within the context of menopause, these stories hold a transformative power, capable of healing not just the individual who shares but also those who listen. This section explores the multifaceted benefits of storytelling, providing insights into how your menopause narrative can become a source of strength, connection, and understanding.

Finding Your Voice

The expression of your menopause story can take many forms, each offering a unique pathway to connection and understanding. Some may find solace in writing blog posts, articles, or even books that delve into the minutiae of their menopause experience. Others might discover their voice through speaking in intimate gatherings, support group meetings, or larger platforms such as workshops and conferences. And those who communicate best through art, painting, photography, or crafting can find those serve as powerful mediums to convey the emotional landscape of menopause.

- Writing: Start a journal or blog to chronicle your menopause experience. Consider submitting articles to women's health publications or websites to reach a wider audience.
- Speaking: Share your story at support group meetings or offer to speak at health and wellness events. Recording a podcast or video series is also a modern avenue to reach those who need to hear your story.
- Artistic Expression: Use your creativity to depict your menopause experience through art. Organize an exhibition or share your work online to inspire conversations and connections.

Creating Safe Spaces for Sharing

Cultivating environments where stories can be shared without fear of judgment or dismissal is crucial. These physical or virtual spaces should embody empathy, respect, and confidentiality principles, encouraging open and honest dialogue. Here are some tips for creating such environments.

- Online Forums and Social Media: Moderate discussions to ensure they remain respectful and supportive. Establish clear guidelines that promote a positive, inclusive atmosphere.
- In-Person Gatherings: Set the tone by establishing ground rules emphasizing listening without interruption, respecting confidentiality, and withholding judgment.
- Artistic Venues: When sharing through art, choose venues or platforms that align to foster connection and understanding. Provide context for the artwork to facilitate deeper engagement and dialogue.

In fostering these spaces, we provide a platform for individual stories and contribute to a collective narrative that demystifies menopause, breaking down barriers of silence and stigma. In the sharing and receiving of stories, it's here that we find common ground, drawing strength from our shared humanity and forging bonds that transcend the individual experience. Through story-telling, we not only navigate the emotional landscape of menopause with greater ease but also pave the way for future generations to approach this phase of life with confidence, armed with the knowledge and understanding that comes from a chorus of voices united in their diversity.

5.4 NAVIGATING RELATIONSHIPS DURING MENOPAUSE

The ebb and flow of menopause can touch every corner of our lives, but perhaps nowhere are its effects more keenly felt than in our relationships. As our bodies and emotions change significantly, the dynamics within our partnerships, friendships, and family structures may shift, calling for a renewed approach to communication, intimacy, and support. This section delves into the art of maintaining and strengthening these essential bonds during a period of transformation.

Communication Is Key

In any strong relationship, openness and honesty form the bridge over which understanding and empathy can travel. Yet, discussing menopause and its myriad effects can sometimes feel daunting. Cultivating an environment where such conversations are possible and welcome is crucial.

- Start with the basics. A simple explanation of menopause can demystify the process, opening the door to deeper discussions.
- Share your feelings and experiences without mincing words. Let your loved ones know if hot flashes keep you up at night or if mood swings make days unpredictable.
- Encourage questions. Your partner, friends, or family members may need guidance on how to support you. Clarifying what you need can help them be there for you.

This open line of communication serves as the foundation upon which understanding is built, ensuring that those around you can grasp, even if not fully comprehend, what you're experiencing. I found that communicating with dignity helps not only me, but everyone involved. I discovered this initially because I was so whiny I got tired of myself. Dignity became a medicine for my self-pity. In my experience, I can have wisdom or be a victim; it's one or the other, and the choice is clear.

Setting Boundaries

Menopause can sometimes amplify stress, making it more critical than ever to establish healthy boundaries. These boundaries enable us to conserve energy, manage stress, and maintain our well-being.

- Identify your limits. Recognize situations or demands contributing to stress and clearly communicate your need to step back or say no.
- Prioritize self-care. Make it clear that taking time for yourself isn't selfish but necessary for your health and well-being.
- Respect your emotional space. If you need time to process your feelings or be alone, ensure your loved ones understand and respect this need.

Boundaries aren't barriers but rather the safe perimeters within which relationships flourish. They protect our emotional and physical space, allowing us to engage with others from a place of strength and balance.

I was surprised to discover that some friends were nourishing to be with while others were exhausting. I had to make clear choices about who I spent my time with because there were no extra reserves to act as a buffer. It became clear that my deciding factor is whether I feel nourished by a person or an activity, and if not, it's a no. I've made peace with this boundary.

5.5 SELF-CARE + SELF-ACCEPTANCE = SELF-LOVE: NURTURING THE SOUL

In the heart of our lives, where responsibilities often eclipse personal needs, self-care tends to be relegated to the background, viewed through a narrow lens of sporadic indulgences. We relegate self-care to our to-do list, such as "get nails done" or "get a massage." While there's nothing wrong with those self-care items, it's important not to turn them into substitutes for learning about and tending to the inner terrain that opens to us during this time of life.

As we navigate the shifts brought on by menopause, expanding our understanding of self-care becomes not just beneficial but necessary. It evolves into a holistic practice encompassing the entirety of our being—body, mind, and spirit—offering sustenance and rejuvenation far beyond the surface.

Self-care, in its true essence, is about creating a personal sanctuary that supports our well-being, especially during times of change and chiefly from the inside out, not the other way around. It invites us to tune into our bodies, listen to our emotional needs, and connect with our spiritual selves, crafting a personalized plan that brings harmony and balance. This plan, unique to each individual, becomes a roadmap to wellness, guiding us through the fluctuations of menopause with a sense of groundedness and care.

When the self-care piece is tended first, everything in these pages becomes more accessible and fruitful. The biggest hurdle for every woman is giving herself permission and making a "full yes" decision to tend to this first and keep cultivating it. Then, choose this day after day until it feels natural. For the record, keeping our cup full IS our natural state. You, everyone around you, and all of life benefit from this continuous choice.

Embracing Self-Acceptance

In a society that often equates value with youth and productivity, menopause can trigger feelings of insecurity and self-doubt. This is where the cultivation of self-acceptance becomes a radical act of defiance and healing. Self-acceptance is about embracing yourself, changes, and all, as well as recognizing your worth independent of societal expectations. It's about speaking to yourself with kindness, celebrating your strengths, and offering yourself the same compassion and understanding as you would a dear friend. With enough self-acceptance practice, we can begin to tap into self-love.

- Challenge Negative Self-Talk: Be mindful of critical inner dialogue and replace it with internal conversations reinforcing your values and strengths.
- Honor Your Needs: Listen to what your body and mind need, whether it's rest, movement, nourishment, or connection, and make these needs a priority.
- Practice tuning into the Light of your being, which lives in every cell. This Light is intelligent, whole, all-knowing, and happens to be personal medicine.
- Celebrate Your Journey: Acknowledge the wisdom and experience you've gained over the years, viewing menopause not as an ending but as a transition into a new, empowered phase of life.

Practices That Nourish the Soul

Several practices can serve as pillars of self-care, offering ways to nurture your well-being on a deep, soulful level.

- Meditation: Whether guided or silent, meditation provides a space for stillness and connection, helping to calm the mind and ease the stresses of menopause. While there are many ways to meditate, the end game is to settle oneself enough to connect with your Higher Self, the Presence of

Life that resides inside and around you. It's a whole anatomy of the Self we haven't learned about, yet it is worthy of your attention.

- Journaling: Writing offers a way to explore your thoughts and feelings as a tool for reflection, insight, and posing inquiries to your heart.
- Nature Walks: Time spent in nature can be incredibly healing. It offers peace and reminds us of the world's beauty, regenerative capacity, and continuity.
- Creative Arts: Engaging in creative activities such as drawing, crafting, or playing music allows for self-expression and can be a powerful outlet for emotions and experiences.

Each of these practices invites you to turn inward, offering a moment of pause in the hustle of daily life and providing a pathway to inner peace and rejuvenation. Watching a woman go from a miserable stagnant pool to a joyful, flowing river is incredibly satisfying. If you can't quite tap into the feeling of joy, consider finding a happily flowing river to stand by or in and invite that feeling in. Or stand with your back against a tree and feel the stability. Nature generously shares her secrets.

As we wrap up this exploration of self-care and self-love, remember that menopause presents an opportunity to reconnect with yourself on a deeper level, honor your journey, and nurture your well-being with intention and compassion. By acknowledging the biological roots of our emotions and adopting strategies for stability, we can find our calm center in the storm. These practices of care and love are not just strategies for navigating menopause but gifts to yourself, affirmations of your worth, and resilience. As we move forward, let these insights illuminate the path, guiding you toward a place of balance where the journey through menopause becomes not just manageable but enriching, a testament to the strength and grace within you.

CHAPTER 6

AWAKENING THE SACRED
WITHIN

I magine standing at the ocean's edge at dawn, the sky shifting colors as the sun promises to rise. In this moment, you're not just witnessing the day's beginning but also feeling a more profound shift within yourself. The vast and ever-changing ocean mirrors the transformative power of menopause—a time that invites adaptation and a profound spiritual awakening.

Menopause invites us to explore the deeper currents of our being. It's an opening to connect with wisdom that has always been there, whispering to us, waiting to be fully acknowledged and embraced. This phase offers a unique opportunity to recalibrate our inner compass and align more closely with our true essence and the universe's rhythmic cycles.

"Gravity and wrinkles are fine with me. They're a small price to pay for the new wisdom inside my head and my heart."

— DREW BARRYMORE

6.1 THE SPIRITUAL DIMENSION OF MENOPAUSE

Menopause isn't merely a series of physical changes; it's a beacon for spiritual growth. It's a sacred journey. Shedding the menstrual cycle can be viewed as shedding old layers, beliefs, and patterns that no longer serve. Many women think there's something wrong with them when old energy comes up, but it's the opposite. When things get our attention, that energy is ready to be released. We release the old to make room for fresh and new energy or life force. This time can serve as a catalyst for exploring what spirituality means to you, whether connecting with nature, diving into meditation, or rediscovering rituals that ground and uplift.

- Nature walks during different times of the day can help attune to the Earth's cycles, reflecting on the changes and constants in life.
- Daily meditation can foster a deepened connection to oneself and the universe, providing clarity and peace amid change.
- Fostering a connection with your Higher Self enriches your mind, body, and life in deeply sacred and meaningful ways. It's an essential component, akin to a vital ingredient, completing the recipe of existence on multiple levels.

Connecting with Inner Wisdom

The whispers of intuition often grow louder during menopause, guiding us toward our core to a still point of peace. This inner wisdom, accumulated over years of experience, suddenly finds a clearer channel of expression. It's about listening, truly listening, to the gut feelings, the dreams that visit in the night, and the quiet voice within that knows the way. Inner wisdom is part of the feminine aspect of life, and this particular time in life is about coming into a greater connection with this part of yourself. Even if you feel like you're currently in a tornado, there is an eye to this storm, and when you put your awareness on the eye, the still point, your guidance and wisdom increases, and you can weather the storm with grace.

- Keep a dream journal by the bed to jot down thoughts and visions from the night, which can reveal messages from the subconscious.
- As mentioned, keeping a journal is a personal way to capture essential nudges, inquiries, and insights.
- A creative sketchbook is a way to journal with color and creativity.
- Set aside quiet time each day to sit with oneself, asking and listening for guidance on any aspect of life needing attention.

Light or Tight

This is a particular way of accessing embodied wisdom and guidance. If a decision feels tight in and around your gut area, it's a no. If it feels light in the same location, it would be more likely to serve you than not. I recommend you practice this to discern your unique sensations of "light" and "tight." Start with inconsequential things such as what color underwear to wear or which way to go to the grocery store. When you can tell the difference between light and tight in your body, apply it to a next-level decision. This practice has never failed me. The only way I get myself in trouble is when I let my head talk me out of the embodied wisdom; then, there's some cleanup.

This works because the wisdom and guidance come from your whole Self, not just your head. Your whole Self, which includes your Higher Self, has a broader scope of the components involved (people, timing, highest good, etc.), whereas your head usually refers to your past. Play with it, and you'll see.

Not connecting with inner wisdom and guidance is a recipe for being on stormy seas without sails or a solid mast. The mast is your core and center, and the sails are your way of capturing Life Force. Connection with your Higher Self, Inner Wisdom, and Guidance helps get you a smoother sail with all elements (wind, water, earth, fire, wood) working harmoniously. It's a key ingredient in moving through menopause with grace.

Lessons from the Menopausal Journey

While every woman's experience with menopause is unique, common currents run through these stories, offering lessons of resilience, transformation, and the beauty of change. Reflecting on these lessons enriches personal growth and serves as a beacon for others navigating this sea of change. If one person can do something, any other person can.

- Claiming your beauty, blessings, and bounty activates an increase in them. Notice, honor, and celebrate your beauty, blessings, and bounty in your journaling, giving them a place to be held and remembered.
- Sharing these reflections in a trusted circle can foster connection and collective wisdom, highlighting the shared and individual aspects of the menopause experience.

Embracing Change as Transformation

Change, the only constant, is often met with resistance. If I were to pick the worst offender for a smooth transition, I would say it's resistance, yet menopause invites a reframe: to see change not as loss but as transformation. A woman in menopause curating her transformation is engaging in modern-day alchemy. It's a shedding of the old to make way for new growth, new ways of being in the world, and new opportunities to align with one's deepest desires and truths.

- Creating a ritual to mark this transition, such as planting a garden, taking on a new hobby, or writing a letter to oneself, can honor the changes and set intentions for this next phase.
- Engaging in activities or hobbies that have previously called to you but have never been pursued can now be embraced as an expression of the self's unfolding layers.

Here are some short takeaways from the journeys of other women:

"Even though the changes were not anything I ever wanted, they forced me to accept this new version of myself, and I love her. I know how to honestly love myself now!"

"It felt like I was constantly mourning the loss of who I used to be, but I kept thinking, if I'm still here, there must be a reason. Small gratitudes and celebrations helped me stop mourning and eventually feel better than ever."

"The idea that I had to modify things to 'suit my age' made me angry. I wasn't ready to slow down, but as I made adjustments, I realized I wasn't really slowing down. I was 'rearranging', and the new arrangements suit me so well now."

"The constant battle with my body and mind was exhausting. I just wanted to feel normal again. It felt like I had tried everything. What I didn't know to try was to invite my Sacred Self to the party. Once I did, everything changed for the better!"

"I'm so grateful that Laurie let me 'borrow' her wisdom until I could trust my own; that has been priceless to me."

As we stand at the shoreline, it becomes clear that menopause is much more than a physical transition. It's a spiritual journey, inviting us to dive deep into our inner and Sacred Self, to listen to the wisdom that whispers within the waves, and to embrace the transformative power of change. With each step, we awaken more fully to ourselves, discovering a wellspring of strength, insight, and connection that guides us forward. This is the gift of menopause— a sacred opening to the divine within, calling us to explore, grow, and shine.

6.2 THE DIVINE FEMININE: RECONNECTING WITH YOUR EMBODIED PRESENCE

The concept of the divine feminine is as ancient as the Earth itself, yet for many, it remains a hidden treasure, waiting to be rediscovered in the depths of our being. This powerful and nurturing energy offers a wellspring of qualities such as intuition, creativity, connectedness, and wholeness—attributes that flourish naturally within us but may be overlooked in the hustle of daily life. As we move through the waves of menopause, we're presented with a unique opportunity to reconnect with this sacred aspect of ourselves, to honor and express the full spectrum of our feminine self as a harmonious balance to our masculine self.

Understanding the Divine Feminine

To grasp the essence of the divine feminine, recognize it as the Life Force connecting all creation. Societal definitions of femininity don't confine this energy but is instead a universal principle that transcends gender, embodying existence's nurturing, intuitive, and creative aspects. Its relevance during menopause and aging becomes profoundly clear as we peel away layers of external expectation, cultural programming, and learned beliefs, finding ourselves more attuned to the depths of our inner life and wisdom.

The feminine aspect of life is the same as yin, spirit, and matter (mater or mother) and is meant to harmonize with the masculine aspect of life, which completes the yin/yang, love/light, and alpha/omega wholeness. As humans, we are microcosms—smaller versions, but the same as the macrocosm or the whole universe.

Many of us were raised in the West, which has been masculine dominant for centuries; those in Western cultures are well-prac-ticed with our masculine energy or aspect. Now is the time in human consciousness to develop our feminine aspect for optimal balance.

I recall asking the feminine facet of life to teach me this balance. And she did and continues to. I've even thought that I must have incarnated to be a menopausal woman at this particular time in human consciousness to do this exact work, to awaken the "other half" to fully express wholeness.

"Women hold up half the sky," a quote by Chinese Communist Party chairman Mao Zedong, was true during their cultural revo-lution, is true today, and will never not be true.

- The divine feminine thrives on connection—connection to the self, others, and the natural world, encouraging us to live in harmony with the cycles of life.
- The divine feminine exists AS your body and every other body. Matter is sacred, and our bodies are fashioned from the matter of Earth and the cosmic forces. The word matter is derived from the Latin word mater, meaning mother. We are held together by matter or mother. That's a mic drop.
- It champions our embodied intuition, guidance, wholeness, and wisdom as our guiding light, a source of inner knowing that leads us toward authenticity and self-trust.

It's not a matter of whether you have these capacities because you *are* them; it's a matter of cultivating them in the face of a lifetime of opposing programming and DNA that carries oppression. All it takes is your attention and willingness to choose it and set aside the autopilot habit of relying primarily on your overdeveloped masculine energy, such as over-caring about productivity, operating from the head more than the heart, pushing yourself to do and be more according to external standards, and not keeping your own cup full.

What happens at midlife is the empty cup, and the constant scraping at the bottom of the barrel becomes glaringly apparent. You may notice that worry, doubt, anxiety, fear, and feeling not enough have taken up the space where divinity, ease, peace, self-worth, trust, and creative expression are meant to live.

In this era of shared awareness, we're urged to lay down our weapons of fear, worry, and anxiety, step away from the battle-field, and walk ourselves home to wholeness. Every woman gets to make this choice, and now is the best time to do it. There are women in parts of the world who can't have conversations like this, who don't have a choice, and who suffer their whole lives without the kind of freedoms we enjoy. We have so much freedom we can wail at our plight for the remainder of our days. I'm not suggesting that; in fact, the opposite. I hope the point is clear—we have freedom and choice. It's my honor and responsibility to use these freedoms and choices wisely to do my best to live in wholeness because I know that every serving choice, I make affects the collective. If one sister across the globe benefits from my choice to plant a flower rather than whine about how I don't feel like it because my joints ache, honestly, that's motivating to me.

Not to mention, I feel good in my body almost every day and can show up for family, friends, clients, and life. I can say that in my experience, the practice of choosing connection, creating, being in nature, moving, spaciousness, staying present, and, dare we say, tapping into moments of joy outweighs the prior decades of choosing to push, over-give, overdo, and tolerate too much stress. We were like a fish swimming in the only water it knows. And now we know there are other waters.

Embodiment Practices

Reconnecting with the divine feminine invites us to embody its qualities through practices that encourage self-expression, grounding, and joy. Dance, yoga, and ritual are powerful pathways to this end.

- **Dance** allows the body to move freely, guided by our internal rhythms and emotions. It's a celebration of movement, where every gesture expresses our innermost feelings and stories.

- **Yoga** offers strength and flexibility, teaching us to easily balance effort. We align our physical and energetic bodies through poses and breathwork, cultivating a sense of peace and presence.
- **Deep Breath** is key in instantly connecting you to your Self. Breath is a cosmic life force and is sacred. Our attention to drawing breath and directing it to tight, contracted, or painful areas is medicine. It takes so little time and returns so much.
- **Rituals** can be as simple or elaborate as we choose, from lighting a candle with intention each morning to elaborate ceremonies that mark significant transitions. These acts of mindfulness create sacred moments in our daily lives, anchoring us in the present and connecting us to the divine.
- **A Pause** is a surprising way to make a conscious choice. In the nanosecond that we pause, we access being present and connected to our Higher Self, which gives us an ideal option for the moment rather than reacting and operating from the auto-pilot place in us, which is based in the past. This practice cultivates spaciousness within, a beautiful aspect of the divine feminine.

The Power of Feminine Energy

Feminine energy shines brightly in its capacity for nurturing, intuition, creativity, and fostering connectedness. Often undervalued in a fast-paced, productivity-focused society, these qualities become our superpowers, allowing us to navigate the world with grace and wisdom.

- Nurturing is not only about caring for others but also about self-nurturance—honoring our needs, listening to our bodies, and nourishing our spirits.
- Intuition emerges as a clear voice, guiding us through life's complexities with an inner compass pointing to truth and alignment. Keep reminding yourself of and practicing, Light or Tight. This is a way to tangibly get to know your intuition.
- Creativity is the divine feminine language, a way to manifest our inner visions and emotions, transforming them into tangible expressions of beauty and insight while bypassing the mind's limitations.
- Connectedness reminds us that we are not isolated but part of a vast, interconnected web of life, encouraging us to live with empathy and compassion.
- Surrender is also a superpower, but not in the way you might think. Surrender isn't about giving up or giving in; instead, it's about emptying oneself to be filled with the flow of life, the light and love of one's true being, and then operating from there.

Reclaiming Your Feminine Half

In the dance of life, the divine feminine invites us to reclaim all aspects of our feminine self that may have been suppressed or undervalued. This reclamation is a journey back to ourselves, to the parts we've neglected or hidden away, celebrating our complexity and wholeness.

In reconnecting with the divine feminine, we tap into a source of strength, wisdom, and joy that has always been within us. This process invites us to embody the fullness of our being, celebrating the rich tapestry of qualities that make us who we are. Through practices that encourage self-expression, grounding, and connection, we awaken to the beauty and power of our inner goddess, embracing her with love and reverence as we navigate the transformative waters of menopause and beyond.

6.3 CREATIVITY AND HEALING: ARTS, CRAFTS, AND EXPRESSION

In the heart of every woman navigating the waves of menopause lies a creative being waiting to emerge. This period, marked by profound change, opens spaces within us—some previously unknown—ready to be filled with color, texture, and melody. Here, creating becomes a balm, a way to soothe, explore, and express the myriad emotions and experiences accompanying this phase.

Art as a Tool for Healing

Art, in its boundless forms, acts as a mirror reflecting our inner world, making visible what often remains hidden in the depths of our psyche. Through brush strokes, we can paint our joys and sorrows; with clay, we can mold our fears and hopes; through notes, we can compose our silence and roars. This process isn't just about the end product but the journey, a path that leads us through the landscapes of our souls, offering healing and discovery at every turn. Ultimately, it's to know yourself as the work of art that you are.

- Painting and drawing allow for an explosion of color that can mirror our internal chaos or peace. They provide a canvas or paper upon which to express our emotions, with colors and shapes bypassing the need for words.

- Sculpting with clay or other materials offers a tactile experience, grounding us in the present while we shape our thoughts and feelings into form.
- Writing, whether poetry or prose, gives voice to our inner narratives, allowing us to articulate the complex emotions and revelations that arise during menopause. It offers catharsis and insight.
- Playing an instrument or singing can elevate our spirits, channeling emotions through rhythm and melody.
- Working with textiles, such as knitting, sewing, or weaving, can be meditative. We stitch together pieces of our journey.
- Cooking and baking offer a form of creative expression that engages all senses, with the added joy of sharing the creations with others.
- Dance or movement to music can release pent-up emotions, allowing the body to speak when words fall short.
- Tending a garden, whether in pots, beds, or directly in the ground, is communing with Mother Earth, a nourishment like no other. Consider planting flowers, a single tree, an herb garden, or a vegetable garden, each symbolizing growth and the continuation of life, a living tribute to your resilience and adaptability.
- Your whole being is also art—choose clothing and colors that make you feel happy. Choose thoughts and feelings that empower your true nature. Set tables for beauty. Let throw pillows, furniture, fabric, and wall art be expressions of your soul.

Starting Your Creative Journey

For many, the idea of engaging in creative activities comes with the hesitation of "I'm not an artist." Yet creativity is inherent in all of us, waiting for permission to flow freely. The threshold to this journey requires no qualifications or experience, only a willingness to explore and express.

- Begin with curiosity: Pick an art form that intrigues you without worrying about expertise or perfection. Give the inner critic time off, and play, no judgment, just exploration.
- Create a personal space: Dedicate a corner of your home as your creative nook, inviting inspiration and comfort. Even a box that you can easily access in your closet or under your bed can be an excellent place to start.
- Gather simple materials: Start with basic supplies. A sketchbook and pencils, a set of watercolors, yarn and needles, or a journal can be enough to ignite your creative spark.

Showcasing Your Work

Sharing our creative endeavors can be as much a part of the healing process as the act of creation itself. It's an opportunity to step into vulnerability, to be seen and acknowledged, not for the perfection of our work but for the courage it takes to express our truth. However, it's okay if this isn't a step you wish to take.

If you favor this, showcasing your work transforms the personal into the communal, reminding us of the shared human experience that art encapsulates. It's a celebration of our journey through menopause, acknowledging the growth, the struggles, and the beauty that emerges from this transformative phase. Through creativity, we not only navigate the complexities of menopause but also connect with the deepest parts of ourselves and with others, crafting a narrative that resonates with authenticity and grace.

Exploring the intersection of creativity and healing during menopause reveals art as a potent ally. It invites us to actively engage with our inner world, expressing and transforming our experiences into something tangible. This creative engagement doesn't just offer solace; it fosters a profound connection with the self, providing a canvas on which to paint the next chapter of our lives. As we wield our brushes, pens, or instruments, we're reminded that infinite possibilities for expression, discovery, and joy lie within us.

Even as I was doing everything "right" in tending to mind, body, and spirit, this creativity piece—and dates with my creative life force—were one of the biggest needle movers for releasing emotions, discovering myself, and calming my mind. I can't say enough about the marriage of healing and creativity.

6.4 RITUALS AND RITES OF PASSAGE: CELEBRATING THE MENOPAUSAL TRANSITION

In the quiet moments when the sun dips below the horizon, casting a soft glow that whispers of endings and beginnings, there lies a profound opportunity to honor our passage through menopause. This phase, rich with transformation, calls for rituals and rites of passage that acknowledge our growth, our challenges, and the wisdom we've garnered along the way. It's a sacred path that deserves recognition and celebration, not just within our hearts but also within the embrace of our communities and the tapestry of cultures around the globe.

Creating Personal Rituals

Crafting personal rituals offers a deeply individual way to honor the transition into menopause. These rituals can be as simple or elaborate as one wishes, but at their core, they serve as markers of respect for the journey we've undertaken. They are acts of self-care that acknowledge the significance of this time and the changes we are experiencing.

- Consider a quiet ceremony during a new moon, symbolizing the new chapter ahead. Light a candle, perhaps scented with lavender or sage, to represent the wisdom gained. Include precious stones or crystals that have significance to you on your journey,
- Plant a garden, or even a single tree, symbolizing growth and the continuation of life, a living tribute to your resilience and adaptability.

These rituals act as touchstones, moments of reflection and acknowledgment that can offer comfort and strength. They remind us of our journey's significance, grounding us in the present and opening us to the future with grace and anticipation.

Cultural Rites of Passage

A look across cultures reveals a rich diversity of rites of passage that celebrate the transition into menopause. These traditions offer valuable perspectives on honoring this life stage, recognizing it not as a time of loss but as a period of gain—of wisdom, freedom, and strength.

- In some Japanese communities, menopause is celebrated as a release from the responsibilities of childbearing and menstruation, marking a time when a woman can fully devote herself to her personal and spiritual growth.
- Certain Native American traditions hold ceremonies for women entering this stage, viewing it as a passage into the role of community elder and wisdom keeper.
- In parts of Europe, gatherings celebrate the "second spring" of a woman's Life, marking menopause as a time of renewal and potential.

These cultural practices inspire us to view menopause through a lens of reverence and celebration, encouraging us to weave our own rituals and ceremonies that reflect our values and experiences.

Gathering in Celebration

Organizing gatherings or ceremonies with loved ones serves not only to celebrate the menopausal transition but also to educate and demystify this phase for younger generations. These celebrations can be intimate, with close family and friends, or broader, inviting a wider circle to acknowledge this significant life transition.

- Arrange a dinner or women's circle, inviting participants to share their experiences, hopes, stories, and challenges related to aging and menopause. This will create a shared space of understanding and connection.
- Reach out to women in your life who have been open about their menopause experiences.
- Consider including women at different stages of menopause for a broader range of perspectives.

Creating a Safe Space for Gathering

The heart of a menopause circle is the safety it offers—emotional safety to express vulnerabilities without fear of judgment. Think of this as creating a soft, warm nest where members can rest their worries and share their stories.

- Choose a cozy and private meeting place, like a quiet corner of a café, a living room, or even a peaceful spot in a local park. Or virtually if that's the only way it can work for everyone. The power of Life Force transcends time and space.
- Set ground rules that emphasize confidentiality, respect, and non-judgment. This helps everyone feel secure and valued.

These gatherings strengthen our bonds, offering a collective embrace as we navigate the changes menopause brings. They are a powerful reminder that while our journeys are personal, we are not alone in our experiences.

Marking Milestones

The journey through menopause is dotted with milestones that deserve recognition. Culturally, we don't have the strongest muscle in celebrating and recognizing personal milestones. From the last menstrual period to the moments of profound insight or significant emotional growth, each milestone offers an opportunity for acknowledgment and celebration.

- Keep a journal of milestones, noting not just the physical markers but also the emotional and spiritual shifts experienced. This record will be a testament to your journey and a transformation map.

- Celebrate these milestones with small rituals or personal rewards—perhaps a day of pampering, a special purchase, or an adventure you've always wanted to take. Each celebration is an acknowledgment of your progress and resilience.

By honoring these milestones, we give voice to our journey, acknowledging the challenges we've faced and the growth we've achieved. It's a process that fosters self-acceptance and appreciation for the depth and richness of our experiences.

These practices offer a way to navigate menopause with reverence and joy, embracing the changes with open hearts and a spirit of anticipation. They remind us of the beauty in transformation and the strength in our stories, guiding us through this sacred passage with a sense of connection, purpose, and celebration.

In this vibrant chapter of life, we stand at the threshold of vast potential. With the wisdom of our years as our guide, we're called to embrace the beauty of aging, stay active and engaged, nurture our mental and emotional health, and explore the depths of our spiritual selves. This is a time for growth, joy, and deepening our connection with the essence of who we are. It's an invitation to continue weaving the rich, complex, and beautiful tapestry of our lives, thread by thread, moment by moment, with love, intention, and a deep appreciation for the journey. The art of becoming more you.

6.5 THE WISE WOMAN: STEPPING INTO YOUR POWER

In times past, the term "crone" was a crown worn by women of advancing age, denoting their reach into a well of profound wisdom and their role as community sages. Today, while the word may carry different connotations, the essence of this archetypal phase remains unchanged as one of a Wise Woman. It's a period rich with insight, authority, and an invigorated sense of self—qualities that emerge more prominently as one transitions through menopause.

I had to get comfortable with the idea of power. Until awakening the benevolent Universe of Love, the matrix we live within is a push-pull between abuse of power and abdication of power. Divine Wisdom, because I asked her to, teaches me daily that true power is connected to my higher and embodied presence and, from there, taking aligned actions. Power is right action, not abuse or abdication.

Embracing the Wise Woman Archetype

At this stage, embodying the wise woman archetype means recognizing and valuing the wealth of knowledge and experience acquired over the years. It's acknowledging that with this life phase comes an authority grounded in lived experience, a gentle and formidable power.

- Recognizing your wealth of knowledge and embracing your authority can reshape how you view yourself and how others see you.
- Valuing your experiences, both the triumphs and trials, as a source of wisdom for yourself and those around you.

The Gifts of the Wise Woman

With this life phase comes clarity that can make it feel like seeing the world through a new lens. This clarity, wisdom, and a strengthened sense of Self are gifts that menopause brings.

- Wisdom: The insights gleaned from years of navigating life's ups and downs offer a unique perspective that can guide personal decisions and serve as a beacon for others.
- Clarity: There's a sharpening of intuition, a clearing of the decks that allows for more decisive thinking and confidence in one's choices.
- Trust: Years of living teach us that trust trumps doubt. Remembering and tending to trust creates a solid foundation of certainty.
- A Deeper Sense of Self: This period often brings a stronger connection with one's desires, boundaries, and capacities, fostering a more authentic way of being in the world.

"So many women I've talked to see menopause as an ending. But I've discovered this is your moment to reinvent yourself after years of focusing on the needs of everyone else. It's your opportunity to get clear about what matters to you and then to pursue that with all of your energy, time, and talent."

— OPRAH WINFREY

Stepping into Your Power

Now is the time to harness this newfound clarity, wisdom, and sense of self to assert your needs, share your insights, and shape the world around you.

- Advocate for yourself personally and professionally, setting boundaries that honor your well-being and ambitions.
- Share your wisdom through storytelling, mentoring, or engaging in community dialogues, enriching the tapestry of collective knowledge.

- Embrace leadership roles, whether in informal settings or more structured organizations, guiding with the insight and empathy characteristic of this life phase.

Leaving a Legacy

As we navigate this profound life phase, our thoughts often turn to the legacy we wish to leave. This legacy, crafted from our wisdom and experiences, can be a guiding light for future generations, a testament to the journey of growth and transformation.

- Mentor the younger generation, offering them the insights and encouragement that can only come from lived experience.
- Document your story through writing, art, or other media as a tangible expression of your journey and wisdom.
- Engage in acts of service that reflect your values and passions, leaving a footprint that speaks of your commitment to growth, learning, and kindness.
- Keep a journal of your journey for the younger women in your family.

The passage through menopause, far from signaling an end, marks a potent beginning. It's a time when the seeds of wisdom that were sown throughout life come to fruition, offering clarity and a deeper connection with oneself. Embracing the archetype of the wise woman does not mean fitting into a prescribed role. It's an invitation to live fully, authentically, and with the authority that comes from experience and connection to life.

As this chapter closes, we understand menopause is not merely a series of physical changes but a gateway to a more profound engagement with life. The wisdom, clarity, and empowerment accompanying this phase are gifts—tools that enable us to step into our power, share our insights, and craft a legacy that resonates with depth and meaning. This understanding beckons us into the next chapter, ready to explore new dimensions of well-being and connection, grounded in the strength and insight of the wise woman within.

CHAPTER 7

ADAPTING TO THE ELEMENTS: NAVIGATING MENOPAUSE WITH NATURE'S GUIDANCE

I magine walking through a dense forest, the canopy above shielding you from the harsh sun, the cool earth beneath your feet, and a gentle breeze that carries the promise of rain. Suddenly, the environment shifts, and you find yourself in an open meadow, the sun beating down with unrelenting force. Just like this change of scenery confronts you with new challenges and adaptations, so does the journey through menopause, heavily influenced by the climate you find yourself in.

7.1 THE IMPACT OF CLIMATE ON MENOPAUSE SYMPTOMS AND HOW TO ADAPT

Understanding Climate Effects

The climate plays a more significant role than we often give it credit for, especially during menopause. Hot flashes in a tropical environment can feel like being in a sauna without an exit. At the same time, cold drafts in winter might trigger unexpected shivers despite your internal thermostat being on a rollercoaster. Drawing from the wisdom of Chinese medicine, the elements—Fire, Earth, Air/Metal, Water, and Wood—offer a lens through which we can understand and balance our internal health and climate with our external environment.

- Fire represents heat, often exacerbated during menopause. Think of those moments when your body feels like it's in overdrive, warmth radiating from within without warning. Or maybe your adrenals feel like they're on speed, incredibly annoying at night when you know you're exhausted, but your body won't let you sleep. Embracing Fire is part of what is needed for transformation.
- Earth signifies grounding, which the emotional and physical shifts of menopause can disrupt. Whole food, balanced complex carbohydrates, and little to no sugar keep this element strong. Energetically, this element demands we increase our self-worth to a new and healthy level.
- Air/Metal corresponds to change, reflecting the variable nature of menopause symptoms. Deep breathing practices and releasing old, stagnant energy from the past strengthen this element. It's the element of alchemy, wherein metal is transformed into gold. Menopause is alchemy.
- Water embodies fluidity and adaptation, qualities essential for navigating menopause. It is especially important for balancing excess Fire or heat. This element withers without proper rest and relaxation.

- Wood symbolizes growth, the underlying opportunity menopause presents for personal development and rebalancing. This system is powerful and needs clean food, water, and self-talk. Otherwise, it gets sluggish, and pain may ensue. Wood also represents the Tree of Life, a symbol for each of us as human beings. Menopause is a stage of full bloom of the Tree of Life.

Next is a visual representation of the Five Elements, offering a simplistic introduction that merely grazes the depth of their significance in understanding bodily processes and overall function.

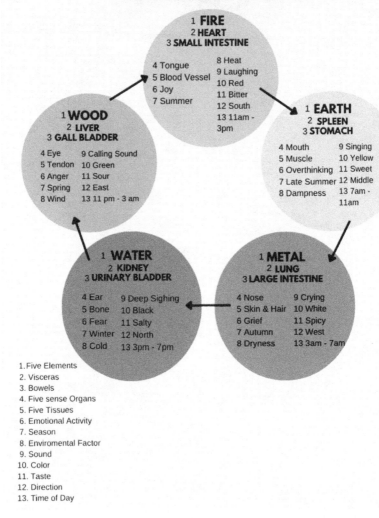

1. Five Elements
2. Visceras
3. Bowels
4. Five sense Organs
5. Five Tissues
6. Emotional Activity
7. Season
8. Enviromental Factor
9. Sound
10. Color
11. Taste
12. Direction
13. Time of Day

Adapting to Your Environment

Making small changes in your living and working spaces can significantly impact how you experience menopause symptoms. Here's how you can align your environment with your needs.

- Use fans or air conditioning to mitigate the effects of hot flashes. Positioning a fan in your bedroom can make nights more bearable.
- Humidifiers add moisture to dry air, especially in heated indoor environments, helping to soothe dry skin and eyes.
- Dressing in layers allows for quick adjustments to unpredictable body temperature changes, providing comfort and convenience.

Seasonal Strategies

As the seasons change, so do our strategies for managing menopause symptoms.

- Summer: Staying hydrated is vital. Carry a hat and water bottle, and opt for light, breathable fabrics to help manage heat.
- Winter: Layering becomes your best friend. Warm socks and thermal undergarments can provide comfort without overheating.
- Spring and Fall: These transitional seasons can be unpredictable. Keep a scarf and a lightweight jacket handy for sudden temperature changes.

Climate and Mood

Seasonal changes can also influence your mood and emotional well-being. For those experiencing seasonal affective disorder (SAD) or feeling more emotionally volatile during certain times of the year, consider:

- Light therapy can be effective in combating SAD during the darker months.
- Spending time outdoors during daylight hours, as natural light, can boost your mood and vitamin D levels, and taking a vitamin D supplement is also helpful.
- Establishing a regular exercise routine can alleviate stress and improve emotional resilience, regardless of the season.

As we navigate the landscape of menopause, drawing parallels with the natural world offers us a blueprint for adaptation and balance. Just as we adjust our path through the forest or meadow, responding to the environment's cues, we can also tailor our approach to menopause, using the wisdom of the elements as our guide. This alignment with nature doesn't just ease our physical symptoms; it also offers a path to emotional and spiritual rejuvenation, reminding us that menopause, like the changing seasons, is a natural, integral part of life's cycle.

7.2 DRESSING FOR COMFORT: FASHION TIPS FOR MENOPAUSAL WOMEN

Navigating the waters of menopause calls for a shift not just in mindset but also in wardrobe. It's when your body demands comfort without asking you to forgo your sense of style. This balance between fashion and functionality becomes pivotal, enabling you to move through your day confidently and easily, even as your body temperature seems to have a mind of its own.

Wardrobe Adjustments

Choosing suitable fabrics is much like selecting allies in this phase of life—you want dependable, supportive, and understanding companions. Natural fibers such as cotton, linen, and bamboo offer breathability and absorb moisture, making them ideal candidates. They stand by you, ensuring that they'll help dissipate the heat and keep you cool when hot flashes strike. Similarly, clothing designs that favor loose fits can provide an added layer of comfort, allowing air to circulate freely and offering an easy escape route from heat. Wrap dresses, flowing tops, and wide-leg pants are stylish and serve as perfect partners during temperature surges.

Happy Feet

Shoes, often overlooked, play a crucial role in your overall comfort. Menopause can lead to swollen feet, ankles, bunions, or plantar fasciitis. Finding footwear that combines support with comfort becomes essential. It's time to reassess your relationship with your footwear. Those high heels, which once felt like extensions of your power, may now feel more like constraints. I consider putting on a pair of high heels equivalent to modern-day foot binding at this age! Embracing flats or shoes with a supportive arch and cushioned sole can significantly affect how you feel throughout the day. Sneakers, ballet flats, or supportive sandals can become your new go-to choices, providing a foundation that keeps you grounded and comfortable, whether navigating the workplace or exploring a new city.

- Consider shoes with arch support and cushioned soles for added comfort.
- Flats, supportive sandals, or sneakers can be stylish and comfortable options.

Layering Techniques

Mastering the art of layering is akin to becoming fluent in a new language— it allows you to communicate your style while adapting to your body's changing needs. Start with a breathable base layer that feels soft against your skin and can wick moisture away. Add a lightweight sweater or cardigan that can be easily removed when warmth turns to heat. Finally, a stylish scarf or shawl can serve as an accessory and a practical layer, easily draped, or removed as your body dictates. This approach prepares you for fluctuations and allows you to play with colors, patterns, and textures, keeping your style vibrant and dynamic.

- Begin with a moisture-wicking base layer.
- Add easily removable layers like lightweight sweaters or cardigans.
- Use scarves or shawls for added versatility and style.

Fashionable and Functional

Finding harmony between fashion and functionality doesn't mean sacrificing one for the other. Accessories become your secret weapon, allowing you to infuse personality into your outfits without compromising comfort. Statement jewelry, bold bags, and eye-catching glasses can elevate your look, drawing attention to your style rather than menopause symptoms. Similarly, investing in a few high-quality, versatile pieces can provide a foundation for countless outfits, adaptable to any temperature or occasion. A well-tailored blazer, for instance, can transition from office wear to evening attire with a simple change of accessories.

- Use accessories like jewelry, bags, scarves, and glasses to add personality to your outfits.
- Invest in versatile, high-quality pieces for a foundation that can adapt to any setting.

Navigating fashion during menopause doesn't have to be daunting. With a few adjustments and a strategic approach to layering, you can maintain a sense of style that feels true to you while accommodating the physical changes you're experiencing. It's about finding a balance that allows you to express yourself confidently, knowing that you've dressed for the world and your comfort and well-being.

I've found my way with fashion, and my little secret is that if I don't feel like I'm wearing pajamas and slippers, I'm in the wrong clothes. I dress for that level of comfort while still feeling fashionable.

7.3 ORGANIZING YOUR SPACE FOR MENOPAUSE WELLNESS

Creating a sanctuary within your home and workspace can significantly influence your well-being during menopause. This section offers insights into making your surroundings more conducive to comfort and relaxation, helping to ease the transitions your body and mind are experiencing.

Creating a Comfortable Home Environment

Your home should be a retreat that supports your journey through menopause, particularly when it comes to restorative sleep. To achieve this, consider these adjustments:

- Optimize Bedroom Conditions: Ensure your bedroom is a haven for sleep. Keeping the room cool and dark enhances your chances of uninterrupted rest. Blackout curtains and a thermostat set to a cooler temperature can make a big difference. Additionally, consider the benefits of removing TVs and other electronic devices from your bedroom. The absence of these distractions promotes a more restful environment, encouraging your mind to unwind and prepare for sleep.
- Rhythms of Sundown: I have found that following this natural rhythm of winding down after sundown is super helpful. I no longer buzz around or do activities that make me feel wound up between sundown and going to sleep. Thus, when bedtime comes, my system has already begun to relax.
- Sensory Adjustments: Incorporate elements that engage your senses in a calming manner. Soft, breathable bedding made from natural fibers can keep you comfortable through hot flashes or night sweats. For scent, a diffuser with lavender or chamomile essential oils can provide a soothing aroma conducive to relaxation. I add lavender to my lotion and apply it nightly.
- White Noise: Consider earplugs, a white noise machine, or a fan to block inside or outside noise that might easily wake you.

- Pain reduction: Natural or over-the-counter pain reducers may temporarily be important to take before bed to pave the way for the best sleep possible.

Any combination of excess heat, stress, noise, needing to use the bathroom, and pain or discomfort can make sleeping through the night more difficult—but not when you have a game plan.

Workspace Well-Being

Given the time many of us spend at our desks, making this space supportive of your menopause experience is crucial.

- Ergonomic Solutions: Invest in ergonomic furniture that supports your posture. An adjustable chair that aligns with your desk height can prevent strain on your back and shoulders, making long hours of sitting more bearable. A standing desk option and an ergonomic keyboard are also important if musculoskeletal pain is persistent.
- Temperature Control: A personal fan or heater in your workspace allows you to adjust your immediate environment without affecting others. This autonomy to manage your comfort can help you stay focused and productive, even when menopause symptoms flare up.
- Personal Comfort Kit: Keep a small kit at your desk equipped with items that provide relief and comfort. This could include a handheld fan, spray bottle with water and a favorite essential oil, cooling gel pads, herbal teas known to ease symptoms, and a stress ball or other tactile reliever to focus your energy during stressful moments.

Decluttering for Clarity

The spaces we inhabit reflect and affect our internal state. A cluttered environment can increase stress levels, making it harder to find peace and clarity, which is especially important during menopause.

- Start Small: Begin decluttering with manageable tasks to avoid feeling overwhelmed. Tackling a single drawer or shelf can provide a sense of accomplishment that motivates you to continue.
- Create Systems: Establishing a place for everything simplifies maintenance and reduces the chance of clutter accumulating again. Use baskets, labels, and dividers to organize items, ensuring each has a designated space.
- Let Go: Decluttering involves letting go of items that no longer serve you. This act can be liberating, mirroring the process of releasing outdated aspects of your identity or life as you transition into a new normal.

Menopause-Friendly Products

Incorporating products designed to ease menopause symptoms can enhance your comfort and well-being. Here are a few recommendations.

- Cooling Pillows and Mattress Toppers: These products are engineered to regulate temperature, offering relief during hot flashes, contributing to a more restful sleep.
- Sunrise Alarm Clock: Mimicking the natural light of sunrise, this type of alarm clock provides a gentle wake-up call, supporting your body's natural rhythms and promoting a smoother start to your day.

- White Noise Machine: A plug-in machine or phone app works well to block extraneous noise. Also good for travel.
- Water Bottles with Time Markers: Staying hydrated is critical for managing menopause symptoms. A water bottle with hourly intake goals can encourage you to maintain adequate hydration throughout the day.
- Journal for Reflection and Tracking: Keeping a journal dedicated to tracking your menopause symptoms, mood shifts, and correlating factors can offer insights into managing your well-being more effectively. It also serves as a reflective space for processing the emotional aspects of menopause.

Adjusting your home and workspace to support your menopause experience doesn't have to be a monumental task. Small, thoughtful changes can significantly impact your comfort and ability to navigate this phase more easily and gracefully. Whether it's optimizing your bedroom for better sleep, making your workspace more ergonomic, decluttering for mental clarity, or introducing products designed to alleviate symptoms, each step taken is an act of self-care, affirming your commitment to nurturing yourself through this transformative time.

7.4 TRAVEL TIPS FOR MENOPAUSAL WOMEN: NAVIGATING VACATIONS AND WORK TRIPS

The world beckons with its mosaic of cultures, landscapes, and experiences, an invitation that remains vibrant and enticing even as we navigate the waves of menopause. However, the physical and emotional shifts accompanying this phase require thoughtful planning and adaptations, especially when travel is on the horizon. Those days of hastily grabbing a T-shirt and toothbrush for a spontaneous weekend getaway are long gone. Whether embarking on a leisurely vacation or a work-related journey, a few strategic preparations can transform your travel experience, ensuring comfort and enjoyment remain at the forefront.

Preparation Is Key

Embarking on any trip requires foresight, especially during menopause, when the body's responses can be unpredictable. Packing becomes an act of anticipation, foreseeing needs, and preparing to meet them gracefully and effortlessly.

- Portable Fans and Cooling Scarves: Small, battery-operated fans and cooling scarves become invaluable allies, offering immediate relief during unexpected hot flashes. Compact and discreet, they can easily fit into a handbag or carry-on, ensuring they're within reach whenever needed.
- Dress for Comfort: Opt for loose, layered clothing made from natural, breathable fabrics. This allows for easy adjustments in response to body temperature changes. Comfortable footwear is also crucial, especially on significant walking or standing days.
- Travel-Friendly Food: Snacks that balance blood sugar levels are crucial. Consider packing almonds, whole-grain crackers, cheese sticks, or small fruit packs. These can stave off hunger and help maintain energy levels without the inconvenience of finding suitable food options while on the move.
- Mindful Movement: Make it a point to move regularly on longer flights or drives. Simple stretches, airport and aisle walks, or even stopping at rest areas to walk can improve circulation, reduce stiffness, and improve overall comfort. Listen to your body, and she will guide you.

- Symptom-Relief Medication: Keep a well-organized kit of any natural, prescribed, or over-the-counter medications you use to manage menopause symptoms. Also, a small first-aid kit for general needs should be included. Having these at hand can prevent discomfort from turning into distress.
- Hydration Aids: A collapsible water bottle is eco-friendly and practical, ensuring you stay hydrated. Additionally, herbal teas known for their soothing properties, such as chamomile or peppermint, can be a comfort during long flights or drives.

With its inherent unpredictability, travel mirrors the menopause experience in many ways. Both invite us to step out of our comfort zones and face challenges with resilience and creativity. By preparing thoughtfully for our journeys, acknowledging our needs, and adjusting ensure comfort, we open ourselves up to the world's vastness and beauty without reservation. The road ahead, with all its uncharted territory, awaits with promise and potential, an adventure to be embraced with an open heart and a spirit ready for whatever comes its way.

7.5 MENOPAUSE IN THE WORKPLACE: ADVOCATING FOR YOURSELF

Navigating the shifts of menopause while engaging in professional life requires a blend of self-awareness and strategic communication. The workplace's schedules and demands might not automatically align with your changing needs during menopause. However, with informed strategies, you can create a work environment that supports your well-being.

Knowing Your Rights

Begin by getting acquainted with your employer's health and wellness policies. Many organizations now recognize the importance of supporting employees through various life stages, including menopause. Understanding these policies sets the stage for informed conversations about your needs. If your workplace lacks specific accommodations, this knowledge empowers you to advocate for them, backed by understanding your employer's broader health and wellness commitments.

- Look through your employee handbook or the HR portal for any mention of wellness support or accommodations.
- If direct policies on menopause support are absent, consider how existing health and wellness policies could be applied or extended to include menopause-related needs.

Foster a Supportive Work Environment

Creating an environment that acknowledges and adapts to menopause begins with open dialogue. Conversations with HR and your manager about your needs can pave the way for practical accommodations. When initiating these discussions, focus on how adjustments can maintain or even enhance your productivity and well-being at work.

- Schedule a meeting with HR to discuss your needs and explore possible accommodations.
- Prepare to suggest specific changes that would support you, such as flexible working hours or the ability to work from home when needed.

Manage Symptoms with Discretion

Even with the most understanding workplace, the desire for discretion regarding menopause symptoms is common. Preparing a personal comfort kit that you can keep at your desk or workspace allows you to address symptoms promptly and privately.

Cultivate Awareness and Empathy

Enhancing workplace empathy toward menopause can transform the work environment, making it more inclusive and supportive. Consider opportunities to raise awareness, such as wellness workshops or informational sessions. Sharing reliable information about menopause can dispel myths and build a culture of understanding and support.

- Propose the inclusion of menopause awareness in wellness programs or diversity and inclusion initiatives.
- If you feel comfortable doing so, offer to share your experiences in a way that educates and encourages open dialogue.

In the tapestry of professional life, menopause represents another thread, weaving through our experiences and interactions. You can confidently navigate this phase by understanding your rights, advocating for a supportive environment, managing symptoms with grace, and fostering awareness. These strategies enhance your well-being and contribute to a workplace culture that values and supports its employees through all stages of life.

As we close this discussion, remember that menopause, while deeply personal, also holds universal aspects that resonate across experiences. The steps we take to advocate for ourselves in the workplace reflect broader themes of self-care, empowerment, and community building.

Moving forward, let's carry these themes into our exploration of planning for the future, where we'll look at how the insights gained during menopause can inform our vision and decisions.

CHAPTER 8
BUILDING YOUR MENOPAUSE SUPPORT NETWORK

I magine a tree in your backyard that you've watched grow over the years. It needed constant care—water, sunlight, and protection in its early days. As it matured, its roots deepened, and its branches spread wide, offering shade and beauty without needing much from you. Like us, this tree goes through cycles and changes, adapting and growing stronger with each passing season. Now, picture this tree thriving, its leaves lush and green, a testament to the care invested and the natural resilience it holds. This is akin to our journey through menopause and into the following years. It's a time to focus on nurturing our health, ensuring we remain strong, grounded, and vibrant, like the tree, ready to flourish in every season.

Many traditions consider humans to be like a Tree of Life. We root into Earth like a tree, receive cosmic life force from above like a tree, and create fruitful and bountiful experiences throughout life. Some seasons are for resting, some are for shedding the old, and some are for gathering enough energy for fruiting. There is great value in honoring the seasons.

What if the season of menopause is a unique expression of rest, shedding or releasing the old, cultivating energy, and then blooming into a new phase of life with a whole new body, mind, and spirit? This is precisely why I love the lotus flower; it grows out of the deep, dark, dank mud of what has come until now. This dense, thick mud is the exact nourishment the lotus needs to be strong and nourished enough to be pulled up by the light of the sun, moon, and stars and become a beautiful bloom. That's you and me, nourished by all that has come before, being pulled up by the light to BE our whole self.

8.1 ONLINE FORUMS AND SOCIAL MEDIA: CONNECTING WITH A GLOBAL SISTERHOOD

We'll put many things in our medicine bag on this journey; support is one of them. The potential for connection and community is boundless in a world where the digital landscape is as vast and varied as the physical one. For women navigating the waves of menopause, the internet offers a lifeline—a way to reach across continents and time zones and find solace, support, and shared wisdom. This section guides you through the maze of online platforms, helping you to forge meaningful connections while safeguarding your privacy and well-being.

Engaging Effectively

Once you've found a few communities that feel like a good fit, the next step is to engage. But diving into online discussions can feel daunting. Here's how to make your foray into these digital spaces rewarding and respectful.

- Introduce Yourself: Many groups appreciate a brief introduction. Share only what you're comfortable with, perhaps why you joined, and what you hope to find or offer.
- Be a Good Digital Citizen: Respect differing opinions. Online discussions can get heated, especially around topics like hormone replacement therapy or alternative treatments. Approach every interaction with kindness and an open mind.
- Share and Share Alike: If you've found a helpful article, resource, or personal insight, don't hesitate to share it with the group. The power of these communities lies in the shared wisdom of their members.

Protecting Privacy

While the internet offers anonymity, it's wise to tread carefully when sharing personal information. Safeguarding your privacy ensures that digital engagement remains a positive part of your menopause journey as you seek support and connection.

Leveraging Social Media for Awareness

Social media isn't just for connecting; it's also a powerful tool for raising awareness about menopause. By sharing information, stories, and resources, you contribute to a larger conversation that challenges taboos and spreads knowledge.

- Create and Share Content: Whether writing blog posts, sharing infographics, or even starting a YouTube channel, creating content about your menopause experience can inspire others and foster a deeper understanding of this life stage.

- Participate in Awareness Campaigns: Look for hashtags, challenges, or awareness days related to women's health and menopause. By joining these campaigns, you help amplify their message, reaching a wider audience.
- Educate with Empathy: Aim to educate and empathize when sharing information or personal stories. Remember, menopause affects every woman differently. Highlighting a range of experiences promotes a more inclusive understanding of menopause.

In the vast expanse of the internet, finding your tribe—a community of women who understand, support, and uplift each other through menopause—can transform this life stage from a solitary trek into a shared voyage of discovery. By selecting the right platforms, engaging with kindness and respect, protecting your privacy, and using your voice to raise awareness, you help weave a global sisterhood. One that not only navigates menopause together but also reshapes the conversation for generations to come.

8.2 WORKSHOPS AND RETREATS: IMMERSIVE EXPERIENCES FOR HEALING AND GROWTH

Specific threads shimmer in the tapestry of life, promising deep healing and profound connection. Workshops and retreats dedicated to navigating menopause weave these threads into a cocoon of knowledge, camaraderie, and renewal. Here, we explore how these immersive experiences can light the way through menopause, bringing solace, understanding, and a sense of shared destiny.

Retreats for Deep Connection

Retreats offer a sanctuary from the daily grind, a space where the soul can breathe, and the heart can open. They invite participants to step away from their routines and immerse themselves in the healing journey of menopause. The benefits of such retreats are manifold, providing relief and relaxation and fostering a profound sense of connection among attendees.

- Select a Serene Location: Whether nestled in the mountains, by the sea, or in a tranquil countryside, the chosen locale should inspire peace and reflection.
- Structure for Growth and Rest: Balance the schedule between structured activities focused on menopause wellness and free time for personal reflection or connection with nature.
- Emphasize Community: Encourage sharing circles and communal meals to cultivate a sense of belonging and mutual support.

These immersive experiences—workshops and retreats—serve as lighthouses along the menopausal voyage, illuminating paths through the fog of uncertainty and isolation. They offer not just escape but engagement, not merely rest but rejuvenation. Through connection, understanding, and the holistic embrace of menopause, they remind us that this phase, like all others, is rich with potential for growth, transformation, and newfound strength.

8.3 THE ROLE OF MENTORSHIP IN MENOPAUSE: LEARNING AND GUIDING

Navigating menopause can often feel like navigating a vast, uncharted sea. Having a mentor during this time is akin to having an experienced navigator aboard who knows the waters well and can guide you through the turbulence into the calm. Mentorship, in the realm of menopause, brings forth a multitude of benefits, enriching both the mentor and the mentee in profound and lasting ways.

Mentorship Benefits

A mentorship relationship during menopause offers more than just advice on handling physical symptoms; it opens avenues for emotional support, wisdom sharing, and mutual understanding that enrich the lives of both involved.

- Knowledge Exchange: A wealth of knowledge is passed between mentor and mentee, from understanding menopause symptoms to navigating the emotional and psychological changes accompanying this phase.
- Support Network: Beyond practical advice, mentorship offers a sturdy support system. Having someone who listens, understands, and validates your experiences is comforting in ways that are difficult to anticipate.
- Experiential Learning: Mentors share their successes and challenges, providing a realistic perspective on managing menopause. This sharing of stories fosters a deeper understanding and preparedness for the mentee.
- Empowerment and Confidence: Having a guide who has gone before can boost confidence in handling menopause, empowering the mentee to make informed decisions about their health and well-being.

Finding a Mentor

If one knows where to look, the path to finding or becoming a mentor is dotted with opportunities.

- Local Communities and Health Centers: Often, local health centers or community groups organize menopause support groups or workshops where you can connect with potential mentors or offer guidance to others.
- Online Platforms and Forums: Digital spaces dedicated to women's health are fertile ground for mentorship connections. Engaging in discussions and sharing your insights can naturally lead to mentorship opportunities.
- Health Organizations: Some health organizations offer structured mentorship programs. These can be excellent resources for connecting with mentors who have a professional understanding of menopause.
- Personal Mentors: Within this journey, some women specialize in various aspects, both professionals and non-professionals, who can offer tailored support that resonates with you on a more personal level.

In the dance of mentorship, both participants evolve, learning from each other and growing in understanding and empathy. With their wealth of experience, the mentor serves as a lighthouse, guiding the mentee through the often-tumultuous waters of menopause. In turn, the mentee's journey and insights bring fresh perspectives, reminding the mentor of the diverse ways women experience and navigate this significant life phase. Through this reciprocal exchange, both are enriched and fortified with new knowledge and a deeper understanding of the power of shared experiences.

I've had many mentors, and I am a mentor; no matter how you slice it, the choice to bring someone into your world who is several steps ahead of you is invaluable, akin to having a guide in a foreign country.

8.4 CREATING A SUSTAINABLE SELF-CARE ROUTINE: INCORPORATING DAILY RITUALS FOR WELLNESS

Self-care, often painted with broad strokes, holds unique meanings and practices for each individual. It's a tapestry woven from physical, emotional, and spiritual well-being threads tailored to one's life and needs. For women navigating menopause, self-care guides them through fluctuations with a promise of balance and tranquility.

Suppose you are a sandwich woman, caring for children and aging parents, or you had children later in life. In that case, it may seem that taking time for yourself is selfish and impossible but imagine showing up for your family and obligations with a cup that's full rather than empty. Imagine showing your children a mother who takes care of herself, making every self-care step you take—however small—matter.

Defining Personal Self-Care

Self-care during menopause is about listening—tuning into your body's whispers and roars, acknowledging its needs, and responding with kindness. It's a dialogue, a give-and-take between you and your body, where understanding deepens over time. This personalized approach might mean prioritizing sleep one day, nourishing your body with wholesome foods the next, or perhaps finding solace in quiet moments of meditation. The key lies in recognizing that self-care is not static; it's dynamic and evolves, just as you do.

Daily Rituals for Balance

In the rhythm of everyday life, small rituals act as anchors, providing stability amid change. Incorporating these practices fosters a sense of balance and wellness, nurturing body and soul.

- Morning Meditations: Greet the day with stillness, allowing thoughts to ebb and flow like the tide, grounding you in the present moment.
- Gratitude Journaling: Write down moments or things you're thankful for each evening. However small, this practice illuminates the day's blessings, fostering a positive mindset.
- Menopause Mentorship: Engaging regularly can keep you sane and on track with choices that make moving through menopause more graceful.
- Evening Wind-Down Routines: Dedicate time before bed to unwind. This might involve a warm bath, reading, or gentle stretches, signaling your body that it's time to rest.

While it can feel challenging to tend to "all the things" during menopause, it's harder not to. Do what you can when you can, and remember, you have the rest of your life to get really good at tending to your exquisite self-care. In the next chapter, we'll mention "bending time."

Evolving Your Self-Care Routine

As menopause unfolds, stay attuned to your body's changing needs. What works today may not work tomorrow, and that's okay. Regularly assess your self-care practices, adapting them to fit your current state of being. This flexible, responsive approach ensures that your self-care routine remains relevant, a true reflection of where you are on your path.

Self-care is a testament to every woman's strength and adaptability. It's a practice of honoring oneself, of nurturing the body, mind, and spirit with patience and love. Through personalized rituals, menopause-specific practices, and a commitment to evolution, self-care becomes not just a strategy for navigating menopause but a way of living deeply, fully, and with intention.

As we close this chapter, remember that self-care is your right and your reservoir of strength. It's the daily acts of kindness you bestow upon yourself, the rituals that bring balance and wellness, and the practices tailored to ease your menopause experience. The more you keep your cup full, the easier your journey will be. This journey of self-discovery and renewal opens doors to embracing life with vitality and joy, readying you for today, tomorrow, and the adventures that lie ahead.

8.5 LIFE AFTER MENOPAUSE: SETTING NEW GOALS AND DREAMS

After the waves of menopause recede, a calm sea of opportunity awaits. This period invites a refreshing introspection and the chance to repaint the canvas of life. Gone are the days of being tethered to the unpredictable tides of hormonal shifts. Now, the horizon broadens, beckoning with the promise of unfettered exploration and growth.

Reevaluating Life Goals

Post menopause, with its newfound stability, offers a splendid time to reflect on where you stand and where you wish to go. Life goals, both personal and professional, may shift in light of the experiences and insights gained.

- Reflect on achievements and aspirations with a fresh perspective, considering what genuinely brings satisfaction and joy.
- Set aside time for deep reflection through journaling or discussions with trusted friends to identify what resonates with you now.

This phase could unveil desires previously shelved due to responsibilities or societal expectations. It's a ripe moment to align ambitions with the true Self, encouraged by the wisdom and confidence menopause bestows.

Pursuing Passions and Interests

With a clearer understanding of personal goals, the pursuit of long-held passions or burgeoning interests becomes possible. This exploration enriches life, infusing it with excitement and purpose.

Navigating Changes in Relationships

As life transforms after menopause, so do relationships. This period can alter dynamics, necessitating open communication and recalibration of connections.

- Foster dialogue with partners, family, and friends about evolving needs and how these shifts may influence relationships. It's essential for mutual understanding and support.
- Seek new connections that resonate with current interests and values. Joining clubs, groups, or online communities related to your hobbies or the subjects you're learning about can introduce you to like-minded individuals, enriching your social circle and support network.

It's also a time for strengthening relationships with oneself, appreciating solitude, and enjoying one's company, recognizing that personal fulfillment contributes significantly to the richness of other relationships.

Planning for Retirement

For some, the postmenopausal phase coincides with considerations around retirement. This significant life shift presents opportunities and challenges requiring thoughtful planning. Retirement planning is not solely about financial readiness but preparing for a fulfilling and active life that mirrors your interests and aspirations.

As the curtain rises on the act of life that follows menopause, a world brimming with possibilities unfolds. It's a time ripe for introspection, realignment, and pursuing dreams that may have been deferred. With the insights and resilience honed through the menopausal transition, navigating these opportunities becomes feasible and exhilarating. The postmenopausal phase is a period of profound satisfaction and joy, marked by personal growth, enriched relationships, and the pursuit of passions that lend color and texture to your life.

CHAPTER 9

REAL AND RAW

In my late forties, I had debilitating shoulder pain, worse on the right, my dominant side. I couldn't reach up, wash my back, or sleep. I did everything I knew to heal… acupuncture, herbs, physical therapy, ice and heat, rest, and things I don't even remember anymore. Nothing worked; this went on for almost two years. I was desperate, and one day, I sat on my bed in that pool of desperation, took a deep breath, and asked my heart for help. One of the first things that dropped in was to notice that my heart was in the same horizontal line as my shoulders. Next, I heard, "You're being called to love bigger."

I'll be honest and tell you that I was indignant initially. I had this little quarrel with my Higher Self that went something like, "I'm a loving person; what are you talking about!"—cue whiny voice.

Response: "Yes, you are loving, yet you have more love that wants to fill your heart and life."

"Hum," I thought. "That's reasonable." So, I asked, "Can you show me how?"

Response: "Of course, every step of the way."

So, I set myself up to stay in close connection with my Higher Self and heart, to learn how to expand my heart to hold more love, keep it filled to overflowing, and pour it into all of life around me. This expanded love also taught me how to love every part of myself no matter what. My shoulder was completely healed within a month, and I've never had a problem since.

I've treated dozens of women in the same situation over the years. I tell them my story, and while it sounds lovely and hopeful, they only want the pain to go away. Almost every woman tries everything else before dropping into her heart for the wisdom that resides there.

The hard part is settling down enough to drop in and listen. The easy part is hearing and heeding the heart because it's so real and true that it overrides doubt.

9.1 SLEEP SAGA

In my early fifties, I didn't sleep for four months, not one single night. I wanted to kill myself. I would drive to work most days, crying my eyes out, not knowing how I would get through the day. It was torture. I tried everything—you might notice a "trying everything" pattern! Thanks to my understanding of health and life via Chinese medicine, I figured it out this way: Night was Yin time. Yin is the feminine energy of restoration and calm. I was significantly out of balance with my yin or feminine energy, so I asked my heart what it would have me know about this sleep saga. What dropped in was that I was being called to develop a deeper connection and relationship with the feminine face of life. The masculine dominance that has pervaded humanity for centuries is coming to a close. The Divine Feminine is coming in to harmonize with the Divine Masculine, and She needs all hands and hearts on deck. That was an inspiring call, so I did what I always do and asked to be shown how. Over the next few years, my devotion to the Sacred Feminine aspect of life has grown significantly; I cry when I stop and feel into that.

I now refer to Her as Divine Love, sometimes Divine Mother as the archetypal mother for all life on Earth, and she is good. She's instantly present, comforting, nourishing, wise, and an impeccable guide. It's my job to invite her into my life; I talk to her about everything, big and small, like she's my BFF. We have tea and wine together (well, that's what I'm drinking; not sure what's in Her glass) while I unburden myself, ask for healing, and await gentle, clear guidance. I very quickly learned that SHE was the call home that menopause opened in me; the nudge kept coming at night. I think that call home may be true for every woman. Divine Love teaches me that if I keep my mind, heart, body, and life filled with light, then love will always be present. Light carries love in the entire multiverse; they can't be separated, and it seems more accessible to keep myself filled with light, and love is the byproduct. Now I know love more deeply, and that's the true healer for anything out of balance anywhere on Earth.

Self-Advocacy

In my decades as a health professional, I've observed something important. With its stunning advancements, the medical system also has a weakness that seems to align with a weakness in many women. The weakness in the medical system is that it has lost some of its humility to arrogance. The primary arrogance is power, and the secondary arrogance reduces a human being into parts that can be manipulated with little regard to the whole and natural system.

The weakness of many women is a tendency to abdicate their power and thus become victims of arrogance. It's one of the primary dances of duality, often called the victim/aggressor, victim/perpetrator, or the abuser/abused dynamic. Everyone has aspects of themselves that are both, yet specifically regarding our healthcare, the dynamic seems to be weighted toward women as victims of the more aggressive system. It's a gift to find a provider in the system that treats you with respect.

I had heart palpitations early on in my journey, so I made a doctor's appointment to have it checked out. The doctor was a very condescending man, ultimately brushing my heart palpitations aside and blaming the green tea I drank. While I was livid, the experience motivated me to learn more. I learned a few things. It wasn't until 1999 that the American Heart Association published a gender-specific guide on heart recommendations for women. Until this point, all the research had been done on male hearts, assuming female hearts followed in lockstep, which is not the case. Same scenario with female brains. Much of the research until the late twentieth century was aimed at documenting the "natural inferiority" of women.

I also discovered that the bioidentical hormone progesterone, a muscle relaxant, stopped the palpitations. I was low due to perimenopause, and it was a simple and natural solution.

The age-old oppression endured by half of humanity, often ingrained in women's DNA, perpetuating cycles of victimhood and abuse, is nearing its end. As women, by each of us doing our part, we collectively propel this 'end' across the finish line. Fulfilling our part entails advocating for ourselves and fostering equitable partnerships with healthcare providers founded on mutual respect.

Of course, this requires researching what's important to you, being prepared with questions, and even saying it out loud to yourself beforehand to ensure you get the level of care that matters. If this isn't easy for you, prepare for appointments as if you were giving a talk—practice in the mirror and hear the words come out of your mouth several times privately so they feel comfortable rolling off your lips during your appointment. I've guided numerous women who felt apprehensive about communicating openly with their doctors, helping them articulate their concerns effectively. With practice, they all improve their ability to advocate for themselves at this level. What if we're undergoing a medical renaissance, and your part is essential? It's my sense that we are, and your part matters.

9.2 THE WRETCHEDNESS OF WORRY

I can no longer track how many women say some version of this: "I'm just a worrier; my mom was a worrier; that's just who I am."

And I always reply, "It may be true that you're good at worrying, and that's just because you're well practiced at it, but more importantly, it's not the larger Truth." I'll skip all the parts that involve pushback and cut to the part about asking every woman who knows worry more intimately than she knows trust to practice offering her worry to Love. Ask to be shown an alternative to the worry, such to envision the best possible outcome rather than the worst. I can tell you it works. Worry is seeing an outcome that feels scary. Flipping the script to see the best possible outcome is a much better use of your energy. The stress reduction alone from flipping the script is huge.

A few years ago, I realized that I had this constant undercurrent of "Something is wrong, bad, and not okay," a form of worry in disguise. Once I became conscious of this, I realized I'd lived with it my entire adult life. I began countering it with, "Everything is right and good." I also love this prayer: "Divine Love, thank you for gently ordering my mind, body, and life." And She does, and She's good at it. If I'm regularly emptying myself to be filled by Her, things are smooth and work out better than I can imagine. I've been saying that prayer for a long while, along with, "Everything at this moment is right, good, and okay," which is true in every moment now that the undercurrent is no longer there, and it's pretty liberating.

It seems menopause is a time to root out these non-truths and return them to Love, which builds trust. The energy that is liberated by doing this is a perfect counterbalance to the shit show that menopause feels like without it. Initially, it may seem like there's too much to root out, so why bother? It's too overwhelming, but in my experience, it's manageable if I don't go hunting for anything but rather let it come up naturally. If it's up, it's time, and it's never been too much at once, with Divine Love gently ordering all of it.

Good people, especially women, somehow think their worry will help, and it doesn't. In fact, it hurts more than it helps, especially the worrier. I understand that it's like crack cocaine in that it might take a minute to discover how to not be addicted to it, but make no mistake, worry is no different than any other addictive substance—it's toxic to the individual and pollutes the life around her.

The Bane of "Not Enough"

I have a cosmology for you to consider. What if, on a soul level, we knew the maze of the matrix we were about to incarnate into, and we said emphatically, "Let me in. I know I'll find the hidden treasure. I can't lose!" We knew there would be pre-programmed beliefs and cultural limitations to wade through, such as "You're not enough, you're unworthy, you don't deserve, "This is the standard of beauty, and you don't measure up,' and the like.

There are two things to know about the matrix of pre-programmed beliefs. The first is that the programs are not true. The second is the treasure we're searching for, is love, and that is who we really are. It may feel true that we're not enough, but it's not the real, whole, raw truth.

Yet most of us walk around convinced there's not enough time, money, love, or resources and that we certainly aren't enough. The Universe expands or contracts according to our beliefs. Beliefs are a combination of thoughts, feelings, and actions that we see as the only way things are.

Every soul is an extension of their Higher Presence or Higher Self, and that part of us is already whole, enough, worthy, deserving, and beautiful; it can't not be because it's Life. That's the whole, real, and raw truth. I remind myself of this throughout the day, which gives me access to a presence of self-acceptance and self-love that I now know is impossible to access except through my connection to my Higher Self. SHE knows. SHE is the key. SHE IS love, and I AM HER, meaning I can only be LOVE. You are HER. You are this LOVE. This can only be known and felt by regularly connecting to it in the face of all the programming we believe ourselves to be. I've come to understand that accepting and letting the whole, real truth live in me is my only salvation. There's actually nothing to fix; there is only this to live as. This light carries love; this energy is the only thing that can dissolve the maze the mind creates. How do I know this? Because human beings have been scratching and clawing at everything but this for eons, to no avail.

Now that I live this, I can say unreservedly there's nowhere to access enough worth, deserving, and self-love except in this still point of peace, connection to a Higher Self, and fullness of life. It's exhausting to consider otherwise. Resistance is futile.

Light

Every particle and wave of the Universe is light, which means every particle of your body, mind, and life is light. I am 100 percent clear now that inviting light into your body, mind, and every crack and crevice of your life is personal medicine. Not Band-Aid medicine, but medicine that heals permanently. It's so easy, and it's free. The only reason we don't wield light like a badass is because we've never been taught. I'll repeat it... Light carries love; they can't be separated; it's the yin and yang, masculine and feminine; they can't be separated on our planet of polarity (think sun/moon, up/down, or in/out). As you play with inviting light into your brain and body, you'll notice how it soothes, heals, and balances you over time. Light is the carrier of love, so whole, real, and raw love is your medicine. Go big with this one.

I had a patient who had a frozen shoulder, and she was learning to summon light into her shoulder in between treatments (remember, light is a powerful and personal medicine). After a few treatments, I asked her how the light thing was going, and she paused and then admitted that she didn't see how it could help. I said, "Well, the light is the most powerful force in the multiverse and creates worlds. Do you imagine that It can heal your shoulder?"

And she chuckled, saying, "I guess my shoulder is amateur hour, huh?" Exactly.

Years ago, when I started this practice, I didn't "see" this light for a long time, but I kept doing it anyway because it felt deeply right. Eventually, I started to "see" it, and now I play with it to keep my twenty-five-year-old refrigerator working, to instantly heal a bee sting, to repair a shoulder tendon, or to protect someone I love. I turn to it for everything because it works. The practice taught me to trust it over time because, initially, my doubt would block it from working, like throwing cold water on a fire. Over time, I stopped doubting and started trusting more.

I was interviewed recently, and the host asked me why I thought people used the word "woo-woo" and what I thought it meant. I responded instantly by saying I thought it meant life. Everything is life, and we've been taught to focus only on the cold, hard facts and avoid everything non-physical. The problem is that 96-ish percent of life is non-physical, including you and me, yet we focus all our attention on the 4 percent physical. To the detriment of our whole self, I might add.

Life, love, thoughts, emotions, and consciousness are all non-physical, yet we make fun of certain non-physical aspects and call it woo-woo. I find that to be disrespectful to life because it's ALL life. So, when we talk about light (which we *can* see in nature) but don't always see when we summon it, it's as real as the wind swaying the branches. We don't see the wind, yet we can't say it doesn't exist. I've never heard anyone call the wind woo-woo.

Let's stop calling anything woo-woo so we can include all of life instead of excluding certain parts of life. The only people with authority about anything have lived it; even then, it's their experience. A human wants to live and breathe in all the spaciousness and light of life.

Light is natural and real, and it's the raw material for everything in the multiverse, so until we've tried it, we can't really knock it. If you only take one thing away from this book, I want it to be that light is everything, including hormones, nourishment, expression, love, balance, energy, and, life. I left light for last because it's the most important thing. Because it's the most pervasive thing in the Universe, summoning and receiving it, inviting it into your brain, body, and life, is the most profound thing you can do. From there, all your decisions, choices, and actions will be serving. It's who you and I are. What if it's time to begin living in, and as, the light? Play with it and let it show you.

The Power of Presence

Maybe you're noticing that being present is crucial in navigating everything. You would be one hundred percent correct. Start by practicing being present all day, even as your mind balks, and it will. When you show her you mean business, I promise your mind will allow it. Don't give up on this vital step. Once you've established being present (realizing it's an ongoing practice), you can trust yourself to choose wisely with the inclusion of light, one step at a time.

Only in the present moment can you bend time to work in your favor. It is only in the present moment that you attract the ideal people, resources, and support to optimize your whole and authentic menopausal self. Only in the present moment does your chemistry work for you instead of against you. It's the only place a body can heal, restore, and rebirth. There's nowhere else to be. Ever.

SHARE THE OPPORTUNITY FOR EMPOWERMENT!

You have everything you need to embrace menopause and step into the future with confidence and vitality. Take a moment to offer the same to other women.

Simply by sharing your honest opinion of this book and a little about your own experience, you'll show other women that this phase of life can offer a huge opportunity for growth and awakening, and you'll show them exactly where they can find all the information they need to make sure they're on the right path.

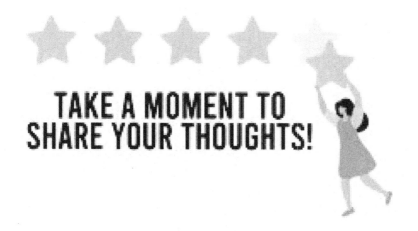

Thank you so much for your support. We're so much stronger when we work together.

Scan the QR code below

CONCLUSION

As we stand together at the threshold of this concluding chapter, I am moved by the profound journey we've embarked upon together. Reflecting on our exploration of menopause, it's clear that this transition is so much more than a series of physical changes. It is a deeply transformative passage that beckons us toward growth, self-discovery, and a renaissance of our understanding of beauty, creativity, and power. Menopause, as we've discovered, is not the diminishment of our light but an invitation to shine it more brightly in new and inspiring ways.

Throughout these pages, we've underscored the importance of a holistic approach to navigating this pivotal phase. True wellness during menopause isn't just about alleviating hot flashes or managing sleep disturbances; it's about nurturing our entire being —body, mind, and spirit. This journey calls for compassion, patience, and an open heart as we embrace the full spectrum of our experiences during this time.

One of the most powerful revelations has been the empowerment that comes from arming ourselves with knowledge, surrounding ourselves with a community of support, and calling in light. This book aims to provide you with the insights and tools necessary to walk through menopause with confidence. Moreover, it has been an invitation to forge connections, to lean on and lift your sisters in solidarity, creating a web of support that spans generations.

By sharing our stories and wisdom, we contribute to a larger narrative that redefines menopause as a period of empowerment and renewal. Please continue this conversation, seek new information, and share your journey with those around you. Your voice can inspire change, foster understanding, and light the way for others to navigate this path.

And so, I call upon you to embrace the role of mentor, advocate, and friend to the women who will walk this path after us. Let us ensure that future generations approach menopause not with apprehension but with anticipation of its growth and opportunities. Together, we can dismantle the myths and stigmas, replacing them with a narrative of strength, wisdom, and empowerment.

Thank you, from the bottom of my heart, for allowing me to be a part of your journey. In sharing these words with you, I am reminded of the incredible resilience, beauty, and power within each of us. We are not alone in this journey. As women, we are unified by our experiences, challenges, and our triumphs. Ready to impart individual and collective wisdom in service of a better world.

As we close this chapter, I leave you with this thought: Menopause is not an ending but a new beginning. It's an opportunity to embrace our evolving selves with love and grace and to step into our power with vitality and joy. May you move forward confidently, supported by the wisdom shared and the connections forged, ready to embrace the vibrant life that awaits you beyond these pages.

With gratitude and solidarity,

Laurie Morse, L.Ac.

RESOURCES

Increasing your energy during menopause: https://sacredhealthacademy.com/
   kickstart-your-energy-5-day-reset-e
Full spectrum menopause support: www.SacredHealthAcademy.com

BIBLIOGRAPHY

Anusara Yoga. (n.d.). 6 Easy Ways to Connect with the Divine Feminine. Retrieved from https://www.anusarayoga.com/6-easy-ways-to-connect-with-divine-feminine/

Anusara Yoga. (n.d.). 6 Easy Ways to Connect with the Divine Feminine. Retrieved from https://www.anusarayoga.com/6-easy-ways-to-connect-with-divine-feminine/

Avogel. (n.d.). 10 self-care tips for perimenopause, menopause, and post-menopause. Retrieved from https://www.avogel.co.uk/health/menopause/videos/10-self-care-tips-for-perimenopause-menopause-and-postmenopause/

Balance Menopause. (n.d.). Menopause wellbeing: how to set goals to boost your health and happiness. Retrieved from https://www.balance-menopause.com/menopause-library/menopause-wellbeing-how-to-set-goals-to-boost-your-health-and-happiness/

Cedars-Sinai. (n.d.). Hormone Replacement Therapy: Is It Right for You? Retrieved from https://www.cedars-sinai.org/blog/hormone-replacement-therapy-risks-benefits.html

Cedars-Sinai. (n.d.). Hormone Replacement Therapy: Is It Right for You? Retrieved from https://www.cedars-sinai.org/blog/hormone-replacement-therapy-risks-benefits.html

Cleveland Clinic. (n.d.). How To Prevent Osteoporosis After Menopause. Retrieved from https://health.clevelandclinic.org/osteoporosis-and-menopause

Daring to Rest. (n.d.). Menopause as an Initiatory Rite of Passage. Retrieved from http://daringtorest.com/podcast/43

Equality and Human Rights Commission. (n.d.). Menopause in the workplace: Guidance for employers. Retrieved from https://www.equalityhumanrights.com/guidance/menopause-workplace-guidance-employers

Executive Support Magazine. (n.d.). Creating a Menopause Support Group. Retrieved from https://executivesupportmagazine.com/menopause-support/

Harvard T.H. Chan School of Public Health. (n.d.). Hormone therapy benefits may outweigh risks for many. Retrieved from https://www.hsph.harvard.edu/news/hsph-in-the-news/hormonal-therapy-menopause/

Harvard T.H. Chan School of Public Health. (n.d.). Hormone therapy benefits may outweigh risks for many. Retrieved from https://www.hsph.harvard.edu/news/hsph-in-the-news/hormonal-therapy-menopause/

Johns Hopkins Medicine. (n.d.). Menopause and the Cardiovascular System. Retrieved from https://www.hopkinsmedicine.org/health/conditions-and-diseases/menopause-and-the-cardiovascular-system

King, D., Hunter, A., Harris, L., & Koenig, C. (Eds.). (n.d.). Dealing with the Psychological and Spiritual Aspects of Menopause: Finding Hope in the Midst of Change. Retrieved from https://www.routledge.com/Dealing-with-the-Psychological-and-Spiritual-Aspects-of-Menopause-Finding/King-Hunter-Harris-Koenig/p/book/9780789023049

Maturitas. (n.d.). Impact of climate and environmental change on the. Retrieved from https://www.maturitas.org/article/S0378-5122(23)00431-0/fulltext

Mayo Clinic. (n.d.). Lifestyle changes to manage menopause symptoms. Retrieved from https://newsnetwork.mayoclinic.org/discussion/mayo-clinic-minute-lifestyle-changes-to-manage-menopause-symptoms/

Mayo Clinic. (n.d.). Menopause facts vs. fiction: The truth behind the myths. Retrieved from https://mcpress.mayoclinic.org/women-health/common-myths-of-menopause/

Mayo Clinic. (n.d.). Mindfulness may ease menopausal symptoms. Retrieved from https://newsnetwork.mayoclinic.org/discussion/mindfulness-may-ease-menopausal-symptoms/

MENO Life. (n.d.). Importance of a Support Ecosystem During Menopause. Retrieved from https://menolabs.com/blogs/menolife/importance-of-a-support-ecosystem-during-menopause

MenoLabs. (n.d.). Importance of a Support Ecosystem During Menopause. Retrieved from https://menolabs.com/blogs/menolife/importance-of-a-support-ecosystem-during-menopause

Menopause. (n.d.). Menopause Mentoring Programme | For. Retrieved from https://formenopause.co.uk/menopause-mentoring/

NCBI. (2022). Dietary and Exercise Interventions for Perimenopausal. Retrieved from https://www.ncbi.nlm.nih.gov/pmc/articles/PMC8828936/

NCBI. (n.d.). Acupuncture in Menopause (AIM) Study: a Pragmatic. Retrieved from https://www.ncbi.nlm.nih.gov/pmc/articles/PMC4874921/

NCBI. (n.d.). Holistic care of menopause: Understanding the framework. Retrieved from https://www.ncbi.nlm.nih.gov/pmc/articles/PMC3555027/

NCBI. (n.d.). Menopause and Sleep Disorders. Retrieved from https://www.ncbi.nlm.nih.gov/pmc/articles/PMC9190958/

NCBI. (n.d.). Nutrition in Menopausal Women: A Narrative Review. Retrieved from https://www.ncbi.nlm.nih.gov/pmc/articles/PMC8308420/

NCBI. (n.d.). Sexual Health in Menopause. Retrieved from https://www.ncbi.nlm.nih.gov/pmc/articles/PMC6780739/

NCBI. (n.d.). The Effectiveness of Mindfulness-Based Art Therapy. Retrieved from https://www.ncbi.nlm.nih.gov/pmc/articles/PMC7171058/

NHS Inform. (n.d.). Menopause and your mental wellbeing. Retrieved from https://www.nhsinform.scot/healthy-living/womens-health/later-years-around-50-years-and-over/menopause-and-post-menopause-health/menopause-and-your-mental-wellbeing/

NHS. (n.d.). Herbal remedies and complementary medicines for menopause symptoms. Retrieved from https://www.nhs.uk/medicines/hormone-replacement-therapy-hrt/alternatives-to-hormone-replacement-therapy-hrt/herbal-remedies-and-complementary-medicines-for-menopause-symptoms/

North American Menopause Society. (n.d.). Relationship Issues, Sexual Side Effects of Menopause. Retrieved from https://www.menopause.org/for-women/sexual-health-menopause-online/causes-of-sexual-problems/relationship-issues

North American Menopause Society. (n.d.). Relationship Issues, Sexual Side Effects of Menopause. Retrieved from https://www.menopause.org/for-women/sexual-health-menopause-online/causes-of-sexual-problems/relationship-issues

NSCA. (2021). Menopausal Women: Recognition, Exercise Benefits. Retrieved from https://journals.lww.com/nsca-scj/fulltext/2021/08000/menopausal_women__recognition,_exercise_benefits,.10.aspx

Rachael Ray Show. (n.d.). Stacy London's 6 Styling Tips for Menopausal Women + . Retrieved from https://www.rachaelrayshow.com/articles/stacy-londons-6-styling-tips-for-menopausal-women-viewer-gets-ultimate-makeover

Routledge. (n.d.). Dealing with the Psychological and Spiritual Aspects of Menopause: Finding Hope in the Midst of Change. Retrieved from https://www.routledge.com/Dealing-with-the-Psychological-and-Spiritual-Aspects-of-Menopause-Finding/King-Hunter-Harris-Koenig/p/book/9780789023049

Today. (n.d.). 5 surprising benefits of intergenerational friendships. Retrieved from https://www.today.com/health/womens-health/intergenerational-friendships-rcna70190

Trocar Supplies. (n.d.). Bioidentical Hormones vs Synthetic Hormones. Retrieved from https://trocarsupplies.com/blogs/news/bioidentical-hormones-vs-synthetic-hormones

Vogel, Kaitlin. Whether You're 25 or 65, Here Are 50 Menopause Quotes That Will Resonate With Every Woman. Parade.com. Last modified February 14, 2023. https://parade.com/1239990/kaitlin-vogel/menopause-quotes/

Women First. (n.d.). Story: Self-development despite menopause. Retrieved from
https://www.womenfirst.com/menopause/thenextchapter/wellbeing/story-
self-development-despite-menopause

Made in the USA
Monee, IL
03 August 2024

63205480R00105